EXPRESSIONS OF DRUNKENNESS (FOUR HUNDRED RABBITS)

INTERNATIONAL CENTER FOR ALCOHOL POLICIES

Book Series on Alcohol in Society

Grant and Litvak (1998)	Drinking Patterns and Their Consequences
Grant (1998)	Alcohol and Emerging Markets
Peele and Grant (1999)	Alcohol and Pleasure: A Health Perspective
Heath (2000)	Drinking Occasions: Comparative Perspectives on Alcohol and Culture
Houghton and Roche (2001)	Learning About Drinking
Haworth and Simpson (2004)	Moonshine Markets: Issues in Unrecorded Alcohol Beverage Production and Consumption
Martinic and Leigh (2004)	Reasonable Risk: Alcohol in Perspective
Grant and O'Connor (2005)	Corporate Social Responsibility and Alcohol: The Need and Potential for Partnership
Martinic and Measham (2008)	Swimming With Crocodiles: The Culture of Extreme Drinking
Fox and MacAvoy (2010)	Expressions of Drunkenness (Four Hundred Rabbits)

EXPRESSIONS OF DRUNKENNESS (FOUR HUNDRED RABBITS)

edited by
Anne Fox and Mike MacAvoy

Routledge
Taylor & Francis Group
New York London

Routledge
Taylor & Francis Group
270 Madison Avenue
New York, NY 10016

Routledge
Taylor & Francis Group
27 Church Road
Hove, East Sussex BN3 2FA

Routledge is an imprint of Taylor & Francis Group, an Informa business

Printed in the United States of America on acid-free paper
10 9 8 7 6 5 4 3 2 1

International Standard Book Number: 978-0-415-99213-8 (Hardback)

Library of Congress Cataloging-in-Publication Data

Expressions of drunkenness (four hundred rabbits) / edited by Anne Fox and Mike MacAvoy.
p. cm.
Includes bibliographical references and index.
ISBN 978-0-415-99213-8 (hardback : alk. paper)
1. Alcoholism--Social aspects. 2. Alcoholism--Physiological aspects. 3. Human behavior. I. Fox, Anne. II. MacAvoy, Mike. III. Title.

HV5035.E97 2010
362.292--dc22 2010007099

Visit the Taylor & Francis Web site at
http://www.taylorandfrancis.com

and the Routledge Web site at
http://www.routledgementalhealth.com

Contents

About the Editors

Anne Fox is an anthropologist and an expert in drug and alcohol issues. She is the founder of Galahad SMS Ltd. (http://www.galahad.co.uk/), one of the United Kingdom's leading substance-misuse research and education organizations. She consults on alcohol and drug cultures for the U.K. Ministry of Defence, advises the U.K. Parliament on alcohol and aggression, has undertaken research with the Home Office and the Youth Justice Board on the nature and prevalence of substance misuse among offenders aged under 18 years, and advises many organizations, including the beverage alcohol industry, on alcohol issues. She has recently completed a PhD in anthropology at Imperial College London.

Prior to retirement, **Mike MacAvoy** was chief executive officer at DrinkWise Australia (http://www.drinkwise.com.au/), a not-for-profit independent research and social change agency funded by the Australian alcohol industry, and chief executive officer of the Alcohol Advisory Council of New Zealand, an organization with statutory roles of advising government on alcohol-related matters, promoting moderate drinking, and reducing alcohol-related harm. Dr. MacAvoy has held a number of government posts in Australia, serving as director of the Drug and Alcohol Bureau, Northern Territory, and director of the Drug and Alcohol Directorate, New South Wales Health; he also chaired Australia's National Drug Strategy Committee.

About the Editor

About the Authors

Billie Atanasova, Australia — Ms. Atanasova has extensive qualitative and quantitative research experience in public health, epidemiology, health program evaluation, and project management and implementation. Her most recent position has been as manager of research and evaluation at DrinkWise Australia, where her work focused on alcohol and health policy and building partnerships with the public health and scientific committees. She has worked for the Centre for Molecular, Environmental, Genetic and Analytic Epidemiology at the University of Melbourne, focusing on the Australian Breast Cancer Family Follow-Up Study, and was project manager and internal evaluator on the Collaborative Care Coordination Project of Emergency Department Services at the Angliss Hospital, Melbourne. She has also held positions at the Centre for Health Program Evaluation (Health Economics Unit) at Monash University, contributing to the Measurement of Quality of Life for Economic Evaluation and the Assessment of Quality of Life (AQoL) Mark 2 projects, and project officer positions at the Melbourne Division of General Practice on the General Practitioners Diabetes Service project and the Increasing Immunisation Coverage through General Practice project. Billie has strong interest in public health, health program evaluation, and corporate social responsibility.

Jean Coussins, Consultant, United Kingdom — Baroness Coussins is an independent consultant, advising companies in the food and drink sectors on corporate social responsibility. In March 2007, she was appointed to the House of Lords, where she sits as a Crossbencher. From 1996 until 2006, she was Chief Executive of The Portman Group, developing social responsibility commitments in the drink industry and promoting consumer education on sensible drinking. Her other previous appointments include Director of Social Policy at the Commission for Racial Equality and roles in education and the voluntary sector. Lady Coussins served on the Advertising Standards Authority, which adjudicates on complaints about advertising in the broadcast and nonbroadcast media, and was a member of the Better Regulation Commission and the Alcohol Education & Research Council.

Irmgard Eisenbach-Stangl, University of Vienna, Austria — Dr. Eisenbach-Stangl is a sociologist at the European Centre for Social Welfare Policy and Research and a psychotherapist and professor at the University of Vienna's Institute for Sociology. She is a member of the Scientific Committee of the European Monitoring Centre for Drugs and Drug Addiction (EMCDDA) and of the Science Group for the European Commission's European Alcohol and Health Forum. Prior to these positions, she was senior researcher at Ludwig Boltzmann Institute for Addiction Research, Anton Proksch Institute, Austria.

Marcus Grant, International Center for Alcohol Policies (ICAP), USA — Mr. Grant is president of the International Center for Alcohol Policies, a not-for-profit organization in Washington, DC. He has worked in the alcohol field for nearly 30 years, first as director of a U.K.-based nongovernmental organization, the Alcohol Education Centre, which provided national coordination of postqualification training on alcohol problems for health and social service staff, and then for the World Health Organization (WHO), where he was responsible for global activities on the prevention of alcohol and drug abuse. He resigned from WHO in 1994 to set up ICAP. His most recent book, coedited with Mark Leverton, is *Working Together to Reduce Harmful Drinking* (2009), which was intended to contribute to the WHO global strategy to reduce the harmful use of alcohol.

Hurst Hannum, Tufts University, USA — Prof. Hannum is Professor of International Law at the Fletcher School of Law and Diplomacy, Tufts University, USA. He teaches primarily in the areas of public international law and human rights, including issues related to corporate social responsibility. His scholarly work has been complemented by service as an advisor to a number of intergovernmental and nongovernmental organizations, including the United Nations Office of the High Commissioner for Human Rights and the Department of Political Affairs. He has been counsel in cases before European and inter-American human rights bodies and is a member of the International Council of Minority Rights Group International (London, U.K.) and the Advisory Council of the International Service for Human Rights (Geneva, Switzerland). Prof. Hannum is the author or editor of numerous books and articles on international law and human rights and serves on editorial advisory boards of *Human Rights Law Review* and *Human Rights Quarterly.* He was the primary consultant to ICAP in developing the *Dublin Principles of Cooperation among the Beverage Alcohol Industry, Governments, Scientific Researchers, and the Public Health Community* and has contributed to a number of ICAP publications.

Fiona Measham, Lancaster University, United Kingdom — Dr. Measham is senior lecturer in criminology at the Department of Applied Social Science, Lancaster University, United Kingdom. She is coauthor of *Illegal Leisure* (1998), *Dancing on Drugs* (2001), and *Illegal Leisure Revisited* (2010), based on large-scale studies of young people's drug and alcohol use, and, with Dr. Marjana Martinic, coeditor of *Swimming With Crocodiles: The Culture of Extreme Drinking* (2008), taking a cross-cultural look at young people's drinking. Her theoretical interests span cultural criminology, gender studies, and the sociology of intoxication, with a particular interest in exploring the boundaries of transgression, the criminalization of leisure, and the problematic–recreational interface in leisure-time consumption. Dr. Measham is a member of the Advisory Council on the Misuse of Drugs, an independent expert body that advises government on drug-related issues in the United Kingdom; she is also a member of the editorial boards of the *British Journal of Criminology, Drugs and Alcohol Today,* and *Alcohol and Culture,* as well as a regular referee for a wide range of academic journals. In recognition of her expertise, she has acted as an expert witness in major trials and as a consultant to the media.

Véronique Nahoum-Grappe, L'École des hautes études en sciences sociales (EHESS), France — Dr. Nahoum-Grappe is an anthropologist at the School for Advanced Studies in the Social Sciences, EHESS, France. She has published extensively on anthropological interpretations of behavior in contemporary society, encompassing such themes as body image, youth culture, and excessive and addictive behaviors.

John B. Saunders, University of Queensland, Australia — Dr. Saunders is professor of alcohol and drug studies at the University of Queensland and Director of the Alcohol and Drug Service at the Royal Brisbane and Women's Hospital in Australia. His career as a clinician, researcher, teacher, and administrator in alcohol and drug services extends over 25 years. He has worked with WHO and acts as editor-in-chief of the *Drug and Alcohol Review* and co-director of the WHO Collaborating Centre for Mental Health and Substance Abuse. He is also a member of the Australian National Council on Drugs, secretary of the International Society for Biomedical Research on Alcoholism, honorary secretary of the Australasian Chapter of Addiction Medicine of the Royal Australasian College of Physicians, and co-chair of the *DSM–V* Substance Use Disorders Committee.

Creina Stockley, Australian Wine Research Institute, Australia — Ms. Stockley, a clinical pharmacologist, is health and regulatory information manager at The Australian Wine Research Institute and an affiliate senior lecturer in the School of Agriculture, Food and Wine at the University of Adelaide. She is an international consultant for the Center for Wine and Cardiovascular Health at the University of Alabama, USA; president of the International Organisation of Vine and Wine (OIV) Food Safety Expert Group; and editorial board member of the *International Journal of Wine Research*. She also served as a member of the National Drug and Alcohol Research Centre's Young People and Alcohol Project Advisory Group.

Betsy Thom, Middlesex University, United Kingdom — Betsy Thom is professor of health policy at Middlesex University (U.K.), with a special interest in social and policy aspects of alcohol and illicit drug use. She is leading the development of a European Masters in Drugs and Alcohol and is editor-in-chief of the journal *Drugs: Education, Prevention and Policy*, published by Informa Healthcare.

Trish Worth, DrinkWise, Australia — The Hon. Trish Worth is the chair of DrinkWise Australia. Prior to entering the Australian Parliament as the Member for Adelaide in 1993, she worked for 10 years in Adelaide's largest private pathology practice, reaching senior management level. During her one term in opposition, she served on a number of House of Representatives Committees and Enquiries, including Australia's International Health Programs and Home and Community Care Programs. When the Coalition came to Government in 1996, she became the first female whip in the House of Representatives. In 1997, she was sworn in as Parliamentary Secretary for Health and Family Services, with responsibility for the Pharmaceutical Benefits Scheme and all regulatory areas including medicines, food, radiation, and medical devices. From 1998 to 2001, she was Parliamentary Secretary for Education and Youth Affairs, responsible for the Youth Portfolio, including school drug education. She returned to the Health Portfolio from 2001 to 2004, with added responsibility for alcohol, tobacco, illicit drugs, mental health, and suicide prevention. Since leaving the Australian Parliament in 2004, she has contributed in a number of key health areas, including chairing the New South Wales Government Alcohol Education Taskforce.

Editors' Note

The phrase "four hundred rabbits" is one of many illustrations of the deep cultural, religious, and social influences on how individuals and communities view alcohol intoxication: The Aztecs believed alcohol to have a divine origin, with a god and goddess giving birth to 400 (meaning "innumerable" in ancient Aztec) divine children or "rabbit gods," each representing a varying degree and expression of alcohol intoxication and drunkenness. Hence the book's subtitle, which at first glance might seem lighthearted but in fact represents an in-depth look at a weighty topic.

Disclaimer

The opinions expressed in this book are those of the individual authors and do not necessarily reflect the views of the International Center for Alcohol Policies (ICAP),* DrinkWise Australia,† or their sponsoring companies and boards.

* ICAP (www.icap.org) is dedicated to promoting understanding of the role of alcohol in society and to helping reduce the abuse of alcohol worldwide through dialogue and partnerships involving the beverage alcohol industry, governments, the public health community, and others with an interest in alcohol policy. ICAP is a not-for-profit organization supported by major international beverage alcohol companies: Anheuser-Busch InBev, Asahi Breweries, Bacardi, Beam Global Spirits & Wine, Brown-Forman Corporation, Diageo, Heineken, Molson Coors Brewing Company, Pernod Ricard, and SABMiller.

† DrinkWise (www.drinkwise.com.au) is a not-for-profit research and social change organization that fosters innovative approaches toward developing and maintaining a safer drinking culture in Australia. Its vision is to create an Australia in which drinking in moderation is acceptable and "drinking to get drunk" is unacceptable. DrinkWise is funded by the Australian alcohol industry, and governed by a board of six community and six industry representatives. The structure of DrinkWise represents a unique opportunity to link the objectives of the preventative health sector, the community, the beverage alcohol industry, and the government.

1

Voices in the Debate

Marcus Grant and Mike MacAvoy

The concept for this book emanated from a workshop held in Paris, France, in October 2007. The workshop was attended by experts from a wide range of disciplines, who met to discuss the terms *intoxication* and *drunkenness* from biological, cultural, and social perspectives.

Why this discussion? How and why people drink are inextricably linked to social and cultural perceptions (hence, the subtitle of this book—it refers to Aztec lore and a divinity-related scale of drunkenness, ranging from mild intoxication, a few rabbits, to heavy drunkenness, 400 rabbits). This book presents a compilation of views on intoxication and drunkenness from various disciplines and across cultures. Separate and apart from biomedical and pharmacological definitions, it is important to understand the broader social and cultural determinants that shape perceptions of unacceptable drinking patterns. For example, although often used interchangeably in the literature, it was the consensus of the workshop participants and authors that the terms *intoxication* and *drunkenness* are not synonymous. Despite the existence of objective ways of measuring intoxication by its physiological effects, there remains considerable confusion about how the two terms are, or should be, interpreted.

In fact, individuals often use their own terminology to describe the state of alcohol impairment, and cultural variations of these definitions are commonplace. Indeed, diverse perspectives, insights, and nuances come into play in discussions about the term intoxication and its true meaning. A multitude of words and phrases are used to describe the behavioral expression of intoxication (e.g., *drunkenness, extreme drinking, binge drinking,* and *controlled loss of control*). These alternative terms have crept into the ongoing discourse regarding alcohol-related harms, alcohol policy development, and epidemiological studies on alcohol and its effects on health. For instance, *binge drinking* is a phrase used to describe a pattern of consumption often deemed socially unacceptable. However, the term has a range of meanings—from a description of a *bender* (a period of usually solitary and uncontrolled drinking) to any consumption patterns in excess of given "low-risk" limits, defined by a health authority (see Chapter 4). Ultimately, the plethora of terms used to describe the many expressions of intoxication proves unhelpful in advancing the debate. By underlining common themes around intoxication and drunkenness and identifying and exploring differences across disciplines, the aims of this book are to advance the understanding of the two terms and differentiate between physiological impairment and cultural perceptions of the behavior they often depict as a uniform concept. To achieve long-term, self-sustaining cultural change around intoxication and drunkenness, we need to strengthen our grasp of the individual and collective meanings and functions of the phenomenon that can be referred to as "drinking to get drunk."

The chapters of this book discuss intoxication and drunkenness from three perspectives: biological, cultural (anthropological and historical), and social. By placing intoxication and drunkenness into these contexts, we can explore their meanings and practical uses in terms of policy development and prevention.

BIOLOGICAL PERSPECTIVE

Biomedical sciences approach the concept of intoxication as a biological mechanism within a social context. By all accounts, there is a measurable physiological aspect to intoxication. As Chapter 2 coauthor John B. Saunders (2007) noted at the workshop, "Alcohol intoxication is a pathophysiological state, a disturbance of normal physical, mechanical, and biochemical functions" (p. 1). A number of official international definitions of intoxication exist. However, there are considerable cultural variations in the use of the term, including among drinkers themselves. The formal medical definition of acute intoxication is as follows: "A transient condition following the administration of alcohol or other psychoactive substance, resulting in disturbances in level of consciousness, cognition, perception, affect or behaviour, or other psychophysiological functions or responses" (World Health Organization, 1992, p. 3). As for drunkenness, the following was suggested at the workshop by Saunders (2007) and embraced by the authors:

> Although, drunkenness may be regarded as equating with intoxication, [the term] characteristically implies the social effects and behaviors that are generally context-specific. There the simplicity ends. … Both terms [intoxication and drunkenness] describe states that exist on a continuum, and both are defined in many ways by cultures around the world. (p. 1)

Simply put, alcohol intoxication is a physical state that occurs after a large amount of alcohol has been consumed in a short period of time, whereas drunkenness is a term often used in a complementary way to denote and describe the behavior of an intoxicated person. However, even from a strictly medical perspective, intoxication is not a clear-cut phenomenon. The continuum on which it exists has been quantified by researchers in terms of blood alcohol concentration (BAC) levels and related "typical" effects of alcohol consumption on a novice drinker (see Table 2.1 in Chapter 2). Clinically observed effects range from talkativeness, flushing of skin, and disinhibition to more serious effects as BAC escalates, including slurred speech, memory loss, stupor, or coma. That said, medical professionals also attest that such effects are not uniform from one drinker to the next. In part, this is because the features of alcohol intoxication are strongly influenced by individual tolerance, whether this be innate or acquired. Depending on tolerance levels, even after reaching a certain state of intoxication, cognitive and psychomotor functioning and behavior may be entirely normal, typically when a person has developed an increased tolerance for the effects of alcohol. So, although there is, in theory, a measurable and relatively dose-dependent relationship between alcohol intake and BAC, the effects of alcohol on motor and cognitive functioning are not always predictable from BAC levels. Numerous factors can contribute to alcohol-induced impairment, including the rate at which BAC rises; the amount of alcohol ingested; the drinking pattern; the drinker's chronic adaptation or tolerance as well as age, gender, and genetic makeup; and individual expectations, perceptions, and experiences of intoxication. Thus, as Chapter 2 co-author Creina Stockley (2007) described:

> [A]n individual's experiences and expectancies about alcohol are also factors that contribute to the intensity of alcohol impairment. *Expectancy* refers to a learned relationship between events and may mediate the behavior or response based on information learned. For example, those individuals who expect more impairment from drinking may display more intense impairment at a certain BAC level. ... maximum subjective feelings of intoxication coincide with maximum BAC and thereafter decrease in a curvilinear time-course. (p. 2)

Our workshop participants and authors with expertise on the biological perspective (see Chapter 2) concluded that BAC levels, although common descriptors of intoxication, are poor measures, and that intoxication and drunkenness are distinct phenomena. These experts agreed that a diagnosis of intoxication must be based on both behavioral (e.g., drunken behavior) and physiological (e.g., BAC) factors. It is the consensus of the authors and editors of this book that the existence of a predictable dose–response relationship is most likely a convenient fiction.

CULTURAL PERSPECTIVE

When engaged in the discourse of the phenomenon of intoxicated and drunken behavior, one cannot overlook the importance of the cultural perspective. Cultural impressions of intoxication and drunkenness are shaped by the social context, symbolism, and perceived purpose of alcohol in a given society, facilitating a multitude of behavioral outcomes (see Chapters 3 and 4). Thus, in one person, the cognitive and behavioral interpretation of a temporary boost in dopamine and serotonin after drinking may result in a calm, euphoric feeling; in another, it might trigger intense emotions; in yet another, it could result in feelings of power, confidence, or dominance. Likewise, a slight befuddlement could bring on laughter and reduced self-consciousness in one drinker, whereas, in another, the same decrease in reasoning ability could trigger high anxiety and increased self-consciousness. So with all these varied effects, how is it that we do find a certain uniformity of drunken behavior within most cultures and subcultures? Arguably, as Chapter 3 author Anne Fox pointed out,

> drunken behavior is in part a feature of culture itself. Culture is an evolutionary survival mechanism that allowed our species to adapt to every environment on the planet. It demands uniformity and predictability of behavior. Everything we do is structured by social rules, even if we are not aware of them. Drinking is no exception. We learn the rules of "drunken comportment" from an early age (MacAndrew & Edgerton, 1969/2003). In essence, our culture teaches us what it means to be drunk. (Fox, 2007, p. 1)

Across cultures and societies, common language such as getting "plastered," "smashed," "blotto," and a myriad of other expressions refers to drunken behaviors (versus a state of biological intoxication). Such colloquialisms also refer to people who may be intoxicated but do not behave in a drunken manner (e.g., people who have "a hollow leg" or can "hold their liquor"). And, although public drunkenness is generally looked down on, the boundaries of acceptable and unacceptable drunkenness are defined by culture. Drunkenness, after all, is found in every society that permits drinking. It may take on different forms, but we can all recognize it when we see it. It can be widely accepted and sanctioned—even regarded as normative behavior in some cultures—or be frowned upon and confined to carefully delineated settings and contexts (these are well-defined and often ritualized "time outs"). In many cultures, drunkenness offers an escape from restrictive norms and social order of everyday life. The French essayist Michel de Montaigne (1575/n.d.) wrote, "The worst state of man is that wherein he loses the knowledge and government of himself" (para. 4); yet, public displays of drunkenness in modern Western society are often fully accepted under certain circumstances, and not only among the young. Older groups are also welcoming of this behavior, as long as it is "appropriate to the occasion." What looks like unbridled hedonism to the onlooker may, in fact, be a controlled loss of control by the drinkers themselves (see Chapter 4).

There is a time and a place for drunkenness in many cultural settings. Culturally acceptable norms can help to explain the range of behavioral effects associated with alcohol and degrees of perceived drunkenness. Chapter 4 author Fiona Measham made the following observation, based on the findings of her 2004 Manchester (U.K.) study, which looked at the behaviors of young adult weekend drinkers:

> [The findings provide] support for the argument that a new culture of intoxication is emerging that features "determined drunkenness" by young adults as part of a broader cultural context of risk-taking and hedonistic consumption-oriented lifestyles. Although this drunkenness is bounded by occasion and location, drinking is often viewed as an end in itself ... with many deliberately accelerating or intensifying their drunkenness by mixing drinks, drinking before going out, or drinking beverages that they know will have a strong effect on them. ... Public drunkenness [in the United Kingdom] is socially accepted—if not expected. (Measham, 2007, p. 3)

For an anthropologist and ethnographer, the concept of "drunkenness" refers to any state of consciousness altered by the ingestion of alcohol. However, the state in question is not uniform. Drinking patterns can be quite disparate, even when they involve the same quantity of alcohol and similar social groups—whether drinking over a few hours during a meal, during the course of a night of celebration, or quickly before dinner.

If one takes the act of toasting and the saying of "Cheers!"—which means "To your health!"—in the honor of a person or an event (a tradition that was probably formalized in ancient Rome), one might ask, "Why is this sort of remnant from a remote period so evident in modern contemporary life? Why do so many people around the world still 'toast to their health,' when many are aware of the possible negative effects of alcohol consumption?" Anthropology and in particular, ethnology can help analyze the contemporary allure of alcohol and drunkenness by focusing in part on cultural meanings to their historical derivative. On this point, Chapter 3 contributor Véronique Nahoum-Grappe (2007) emphasized, "It is important to observe collective alcohol consumption to better understand the chain of events leading to drinking outcomes, the process of making collective choices, and the cultural seductiveness of excesses" (p. 2).

Hence, from the cultural perspective, the term drunkenness *is referred to as a set of behaviors associated with—not caused by—alcohol in a given culture. In this context, drunkenness is the product of culture, societal mores, expectations, and ritualized contexts; meanwhile, intoxication should refer to the clinically verifiable levels of alcohol in the bloodstream. From the cultural perspective, intoxication and drunkenness are not synonymous.*

SOCIAL PERSPECTIVE

There is some difficulty defining at what point the social pleasures of drinking (the invisible effects) and problematic antisocial behaviors (the visible effects) intersect. In the social sciences, particularly the criminological literature on alcohol, the terms intoxication and drunkenness are often linked with problematic drinking behaviors and issues of public disorder (see Chapters 2, 4, and 5).

In most legal systems, the issue of intoxication is considered within the context of criminal law, where the effect or impact of being intoxicated arises in two somewhat different contexts. The first context is when the fact of being intoxicated is raised as a defense to a criminal charge on the grounds that the intoxication affects the state of mind, commonly known as *mens rea*. However, even when intoxication is pleaded as a defense to crimes with "specific" intent (where the intent is an explicit part of the crime—e.g., assault with intent to rape or kill), it is not usually accepted as a justification or an excuse, unless the degree of intoxication is extreme, almost amounting to a state of automatism or insanity, which might be found to render an accused incapable of forming the necessary intent.

The second context concerns the identification of drunkenness per se as a criminal act, with the main issue being whether drunkenness is a behavior that should be criminalized—and whether alcoholism should be treated as a disease rather than punished as a crime. Public drunkenness is cause for punishment in many jurisdictions in numerous cultures. As Chapter 2 contributing author Hurst Hannum (2007) observed at the workshop, "For example, in the U.S. state of Indiana, it is a Class B misdemeanor for a person to be in a public place or a place of public resort in a state of intoxication caused by the use of alcohol" (p. 2). This supports the view, often depicted in literature and elsewhere culturally, that drunkenness is generally considered to be a more extreme state than intoxication. For instance, from a literary perspective, intoxication is frequently perceived as a state defined by internal changes in the consciousness of the character. It is seen as "having a buzz"—a state in which people retain some level of awareness, including awareness of their own and society's inhibitions. Drunkenness, by contrast, tends to be depicted as a state in which drinkers abandon their responsibilities, a form of social (mis)behavior that often carries with it immediate or long-term negative consequences.

From a social marketing point of view, intoxication is a technical word that suggests a spectrum from the mildest effects of alcohol ("a buzz") to the extreme of drunkenness. In this context, although intoxication is sometimes used as a synonym for drunkenness, the former can describe the socially and legally permissible process of drinking, which can at certain levels be pleasurable, responsible, and socially acceptable in both public and private. Drunkenness is the result of intoxication going too far, when self-control and personal responsibility are abandoned, and a negative outcome is likely. As articulated at the workshop by Chapter 5 contributing author Jean Coussins (2007), this behavior is readily described and recognized by:

> [showing] its impact and consequences for individuals; by the ways it is portrayed in TV dramas, soaps, documentaries, and reality programs and regulated in advertising; by the response of police, local authorities, and the licensed trade; and by the nature of news media reporting. … In other words, by its footprint. (p. 1)

Or, as Chapter 4 author Fiona Measham (2007) has noted, a state of intoxication, from a social perspective, can also be assessed in terms of "subjective interpretations of drunkenness mediated by historical and cultural discourses, both official and unofficial" (p. 2). Drunkenness is also characterized as a behavior driven by sociocultural factors, a concept linked to cultural expressions of the physical effects of alcohol, where the context can largely predict behavioral outcomes of intoxication—in other words, social rules and expectations teach people how to interpret the effects of alcohol. Many protective factors can shape and influence the social boundaries of intoxication (see Chapter 5). There is a tacit social assumption that a certain level of intoxication can be positive, enhancing communication and social bonding, but drunken behavior beyond that level may be viewed more ambiguously and as a means to disengage the drinker from his or her moral and social responsibilities. When drinking to the point of drunkenness becomes normalized in a culture or a subculture, it becomes extremely difficult to change—particularly when there exist occasions and contexts in which drunkenness is socially accepted as a rite of passage. Methodologies to change an entrenched drinking pattern to one that does not involve drunkenness have been poorly understood, let alone promoted, and have often focused on manipulating the external factors of supply or demonstrating the negative consequences of excessive consumption, with little effect.

So, within the legal discourse, public drunkenness has been defined as an act punishable by law in many cultures, although it might be allowed on certain occasions (e.g., Mardi Gras in New Orleans or Carnivale in parts of Europe and Latin America). On the other hand, intoxication, measured by BAC level or demonstrable impairment, has been used to define unlawful drinking and driving. Extreme intoxication has also been posited as a legal defense for certain "specific-intent" crimes. From a legal perspective, drunkenness is more often linked with problematic drinking behaviors and issues of public disorder; intoxication is defined as the clinical state of impairment. The two terms are, once again, not synonymous.

The various contributors from the social perspective suggest that drunkenness is a behavioral manifestation of a social phenomenon that can lead to adverse immediate and long-term negative consequences. It is generally considered to be a more extreme state than the physical state of intoxication (at least at the lower levels of impairment). Drunkenness, thus, can be defined as the behavioral expression of intoxication, a phenomenon defined by cultural and social norms, a socially learned conduct that can be triggered even by placebo alcohol. From this perspective, the two terms are not synonymous and the primary concern with drunkenness should not be the number of drinks consumed by an individual but the resulting behavior itself—and its associated public harms.

ARRIVING AT A CONSENSUS

Intoxication and drunkenness exist on spectrums that can aptly be described in both objective and subjective terms. A definition of intoxication ought to take into account both objective and subjective components—from physiological to psychological, sociological, legal, and cultural—and attempt to convey the true essence of this state beyond its most obvious and purely physical manifestations. A definition of drunkenness must be motivated by a myriad of contextual factors and perceived social expectancies. For societies where drinking is permitted, rather than simply condemning and aiming to rid society of drunkenness altogether, our energies might be better spent on responding to the realities of drinking and on working to better understand the visible and invisible effects of both intoxication, on the one hand, and "drinking to get drunk" on the other, to promote optimal cultural, legal, and health strategies for individual and social well-being.

The authors of this volume reject the notion that the terms *intoxication* and *drunkenness* are synonymous; instead, they have explored definitions that take into account the full spectrum of the phenomena. They assert that the two concepts are separate yet interrelated, with intoxication being a state, and drunkenness being a behavior. That said, both the condition of intoxication and the behavior of drunkenness exist on a continuum. The levels of intoxication are contingent on certain physiological variables (e.g., individual tolerance, age, weight, gender, amount of food ingested, and drinking patterns). Meanwhile, the degrees or the extremes of drunken behavior are influenced by factors ranging from psychological expectations to cultural norms and social acceptance (or lack thereof). We also assert that there is a need globally to use drinking as a window through which to look at other aspects of an individual's life, to see how parts of a sociocultural system work in relation to each other. The manner in which the sociocultural system works overall reveals much about the when, where, who, what, why, and how of people's drinking.

This book seeks to draw a better, more expansive picture of the state of intoxication and the behavior of drunkenness. It is hoped that the subsequent chapters—written from biomedical, cultural, and social perspectives—will guide us in understanding these phenomena and help us describe what modifies or exacerbates their existence.

REFERENCES

Coussins, J. (2007, October). *The drunken footprint: Defining intoxication and drunkenness from a social marketing perspective.* Paper presented at the Workshop on Intoxication and Drunkenness of the International Center for Alcohol Policies and DrinkWise Australia, Paris.

de Montaigne, M. (n.d.). VIII. Of drunkenness. In *Essays* (C. Cotton, Trans.). Retrieved December 20, 2009, from http://montaigne.classicauthors.net/Essays/Essays8.html (Original work published 1575)

Fox, A. (2007, October) *Cultural perspectives.* Paper presented at the workshop on Intoxication and Drunkenness at the International Center for Alcohol Policies and DrinkWise Australia, Paris.

Hannum, H. (2007, October). *Intoxication and the law.* Paper presented at the Workshop on Intoxication and Drunkenness of the International Center for Alcohol Policies and DrinkWise Australia, Paris.

MacAndrew, C., & Edgerton, R. C. (2003). *Drunken comportment: A social explanation.* Clinton Corners, NY: Percheron Press/Eliot Werner Publications. (Original work published 1969)

Measham, F. (2007, October). *Intoxication and drunkenness.* Paper presented at the Workshop on Intoxication and Drunkenness of the International Center for Alcohol Policies and DrinkWise Australia, Paris.

Nahoum-Grappe, V. (2007, October). *Drunkenness as a culture.* Paper presented at the Workshop on Intoxication and Drunkenness of the International Center for Alcohol Policies and DrinkWise Australia, Paris.

Saunders, J. B. (2007, October). *Intoxication and drunkenness.* Paper presented at the Workshop on Intoxication and Drunkenness of the International Center for Alcohol Policies and DrinkWise Australia, Paris.

Stockley, C. (2007, October). *Initial comments on a definition of drunkenness and intoxication.* Paper presented at the Workshop on Intoxication and Drunkenness of the International Center for Alcohol Policies and DrinkWise Australia, Paris.

World Health Organization. (1992). *The ICD-10 classification of mental and behavioural disorders: Clinical descriptions and diagnostic guidelines.* Geneva, Switzerland: Author.

2

The Biology of Intoxication

Creina Stockley and John B. Saunders

This chapter provides an overview of the biological processes involved in alcohol consumption, particularly where intoxication is likely. Following a summary of current clinical and pharmacological definitions of intoxication and a case study on legal definitions of both intoxication and drunkenness, we explore the known effects of alcohol* on neurotransmitter systems in the brain, which are responsible for the euphoric, reinforcing, disinhibiting, and sedative effects—all features of the varying stages of the intoxicated state—and on certain hormones that can influence intoxicated behavior. We then examine the intra- and interindividual differences in how alcohol is handled by the body and its effects on a drinker's clinical manifestations. The chapter concludes with an account of current and prospective biologically oriented interventions for the prevention and management of intoxication.

WHAT HAPPENS TO ALCOHOL IN THE BODY: WHERE DOES IT GO?

Once ingested, alcohol is absorbed from the gastrointestinal tract (see Figure 2.1). Approximately 20 to 25% is absorbed through the stomach, with the remaining 75 to 80% absorbed more rapidly by diffusion from the duodenum in the small intestine. It is then transported via the hepatic portal vein to the liver, where some is immediately metabolized (or broken down) and the remainder enters the systemic circulation (i.e., the bloodstream).† Alcohol is detected in the systemic circulation, including

* In this chapter, the unqualified term *alcohol* refers to ethyl alcohol or ethanol.

† Vaporized alcohol can also be absorbed through the lungs into the bloodstream.

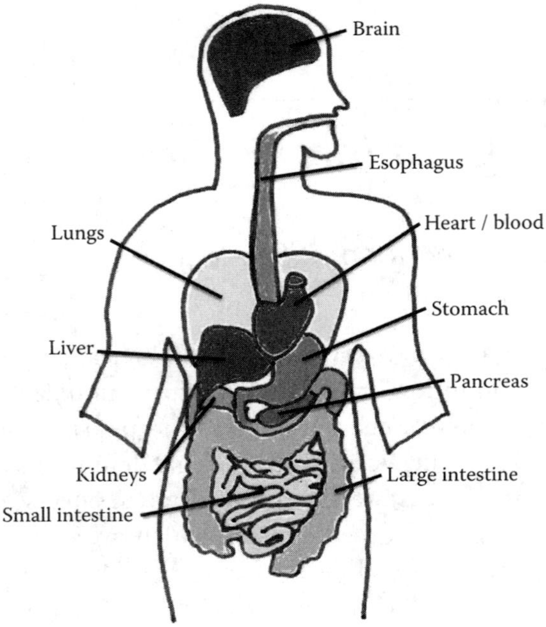

FIGURE 2.1
The main pathways for alcohol following ingestion.

the brain, within approximately 5 minutes of ingestion. A peak blood alcohol concentration (BAC) is achieved 30 to 90 minutes after drinking, depending largely on whether or not food was also consumed.

Water-soluble alcohol rapidly distributes into the total body water, which is approximately 45 to 55% of total body weight in women and 55 to 65% in men (alcohol distributes little into body fat). BAC, the metric commonly used to assess alcohol impairment for legal and medical purposes, is generally measured in milligrams of ethanol per milliliter of blood (mg/ml). An individual's BAC tends to increase by about 0.2 mg/ml in men and 0.3 mg/ml in women for each 10 g drink,* although there can be up to a fourfold intraindividual and interindividual variation in the rate of absorption.

* Although the definition of a *standard drink* or *unit* varies between countries from 8 g to 19.75 g of pure ethanol, 10 g, the most commonly used unit size, has been adopted as the standard definition in this chapter. For discussion, see http://www.icap.org/PolicyIssues/DrinkingGuidelines/StandardDrinks/

Alcohol is removed from the bloodstream through a combination of metabolism (92–98%); excretion in urine, sweat, and tears (1–3%); and evaporation in breath (1–5%). It is removed primarily by oxidative metabolism in the liver (80%) and, to a lesser extent, in the stomach (20%) via the alcohol dehydrogenase (ADH) and acetaldehyde dehydrogenase (ALDH) enzyme pathways. Minor metabolism also occurs in the brain and pancreas. The enzymes help to break apart the ethanol molecule into other compounds or metabolites, which can be eliminated more easily by the body. These enzyme pathways are capacity-limited, and metabolism occurs at a constant rate of approximately 15 to 20 mg of alcohol per 100 ml of blood per hour—or approximately 10 g of alcohol per hour. It is important to note that alcohol is metabolized slower than it is absorbed, and the rate of metabolism is unaffected by the amount of alcohol consumed. Consequently, the more alcohol is consumed, and the faster it is consumed, the higher the maximum BAC achieved. Correspondingly, the higher the maximum BAC achieved, the more brain regions are reached—and, hence, affected—by alcohol. Because the amount of alcohol metabolized per unit of time is approximately proportional to body weight and thus liver weight, the rate of metabolism can vary considerably between individuals; in general, however, BAC decreases by between 0.06 mg/ml (for women) and 0.10 mg/ml (for men) per hour. A larger and heavier individual will have more metabolizing enzymes than a smaller and lighter individual, and so record a lower maximum BAC for the same amount consumed.

In the first step of the enzymatic pathway, alcohol is metabolized to acetaldehyde, which in turn is metabolized to acetate (acetic acid), used in the Krebs cycle forming carbon dioxide and water (see Figure 2.2). Subsequently, a second metabolic pathway, the microsomal mixed

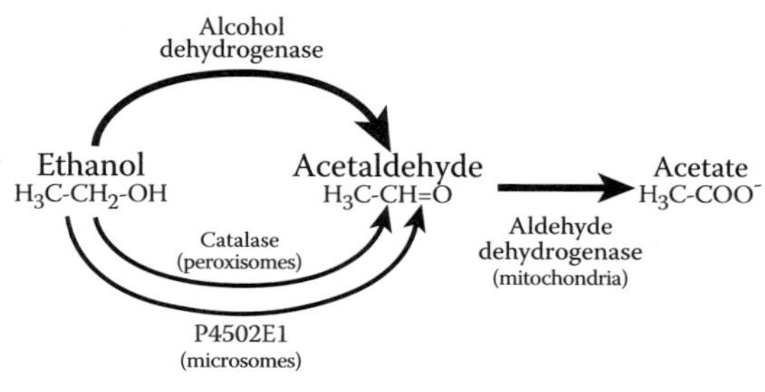

FIGURE 2.2
Enzymatic pathway of alcohol to acetate (acetic acid).

function oxidase enzyme pathway, is activated at a certain concentration of alcohol in the liver. This P450 2E1 enzyme pathway is a subset of the cytochrome P450 pathway that, in addition to alcohol, also breaks down foods and drugs. The rate of metabolism by this enzyme pathway is faster than that by ADH and ALDH. Small amounts of alcohol are also removed by interacting with fatty acids to form compounds called *fatty acid ethyl esters*. These compounds have been shown to contribute to damage of the liver and pancreas.

Competing Priorities in the Liver

Because drugs and foods are also metabolized by the P450 2E1 enzyme pathway, alcohol can interact with other substances consumed concomitantly, such as anesthetics, analgesics, antibiotics, anticoagulants, antidepressants, antihistamines, and antidiabetic, antiseizure, and antiulcer medications. Similar to alcohol, to exert its desired effect, a drug generally must travel through the bloodstream to its site of action, where it produces some change in an organ or tissue. If alcohol is preferentially metabolized by the P450 2E1 enzyme pathway, the resultant blood concentration of the other substance and its effects will be increased, and vice versa. For example, the anticoagulant drug warfarin is prescribed to decrease the blood's ability to clot. Alcohol is metabolized in preference to warfarin by the P450 2E1 enzyme pathway, so alcohol consumption immediately prior to a dose of warfarin raises the blood concentration and availability of the medication and its anticoagulant effects, which increases the patient's risk of a life-threatening hemorrhage. Conversely, the drug isoniazid, used to treat tuberculosis, is metabolized in preference to alcohol. Therefore, alcohol consumption immediately prior to a dose of isoniazid decreases the blood concentration and availability of the medication, lowering its effectiveness in treating tuberculosis.

WHAT IS INTOXICATION?

Simply put, alcohol intoxication is a physical state that occurs after a large amount of alcohol has been consumed in a short period of time. *Drunkenness* is a term often used in a complementary way to describe the behavior of an intoxicated person (the subsequent chapters in this volume offer descriptions of the cultural variance in drunken comportment). Further, drunkenness is a term that conveys a sense of intoxication in a social context, generally indicating a state of incapacity. It sometimes has the connotation of a state that the individual experiences repeatedly and may be given the label of *chronic drunkenness*. In this use, the term drunkenness is analogous to the old term *inebriety*, which has fallen into disuse. Drunkenness potentially can have both positive and negative connotations, whereas chronic drunkenness and inebriety typically indicate a habitual pattern of alcohol consumption that is considered damaging and often socially inappropriate.

In short, alcohol intoxication is a pathophysiological state—that is, a disturbance of normal physical, mechanical, and biochemical functions resulting from acute alcohol consumption—whereas drunkenness characteristically implies the behavior and social effects that tend to be context-specific. There the simplicity ends; these complex terms describe states and effects that exist on a continuum and are defined in different ways by different cultures around the world. A continuum refers to the fact that intoxication is not an all-or-nothing state; it occurs gradually with continued alcohol consumption—from the initial relaxant effects to slurred speech and a staggering gait, and to the extreme of losing consciousness.

Indeed, there are substantial cross-cultural differences in how the term *intoxication* is used and in the significance associated with the intoxicated state (for the legal perspective, see Case Study 2.1). In some cultures, intoxication refers to *any* degree of impairment due to the physiological effects of alcohol. In many Western societies, however, a distinction is made between impairment at lower blood alcohol levels and intoxication, which is defined by a legally proscribed limit or the typical behavioral and physical effects. In other societies, the term *intoxication* is equivalent to acute poisoning—there, the state is viewed as being equivalent to an anesthetic or sedative overdose, which would require clinical attention, potentially including resuscitation. A more general definition for intoxication gleaned from the medical literature focuses on "an elevated blood alcohol concentration …, such that a person cannot function within their normal range of cognitive and physical abilities" (National Health and Medical Research Council, 2001, p. 126). Factors influencing intoxication are, therefore, factors influencing BAC and the cognitive and motor functions affected by alcohol.

Cognitive and motor impairments are the common markers for intoxication (Fogarty & Vogel-Sprott, 2002), often predicted by BAC reached or the number of drinks consumed. There are, however, numerous physiological, pharmacological, and other factors that contribute to alcohol-induced impairment. Of particular consideration are the nature of the task an individual has to perform; the pharmacokinetics of alcohol (rising or falling BAC); and the drinkers' size, weight, gender, genetic makeup, experience with alcohol, and the subjective perception of intoxication.* Thus, because the actual and perceived alcohol sensitivity can vary from time to time, person to person, and situation to situation, any definition for intoxication could merely be arbitrary—as demonstrated by Case Study 2.1 on legal response to intoxication and drunkenness and the review of current clinical definitions.

CASE STUDY 2.1: Legal Response to Intoxication and Drunkenness

By Hurst Hannum

The law is an essential component of the highly regulated areas of alcohol production, distribution, and consumption. Attempts to control intoxication or drunkenness per se through legal means—of interest to us here—vary considerably both across and within countries; as we discuss later, they are often products of enforcement rather than new legislation or official interpretations of the law.

In most legal systems, the topic of intoxication raises issues under both criminal and civil law, and the effect or impact of being intoxicated—drunkenness—is relevant in several different contexts. Perhaps surprisingly, however, intoxication itself is rarely defined in precise or scientific terms, with the exception of specific limits for blood alcohol

* Interestingly, the trend in the 1979, 1995, and 2000 National Alcohol Surveys in the United States was a downward shift in the subjective definition of intoxication related to the number of drinks consumed (Kerr, Greenfield, & Midanik, 2006; Midanik, 1999). For example, intoxication was defined by respondents as having consumed approximately 9.5 and 5.5 drinks for men and women, respectively, in 1979, and 6.5 and 4 drinks for men and women, respectively, in 2000. This trend could be related to an increase in educational attainment (and, hence, better awareness of health issues), aging population, declines in per-capita consumption, and changes in alcohol public health policy in the United States toward lower BAC limits for alcohol-impaired driving (Kerr et al., 2006).

content that are set out in statutes dealing with operating a motor vehicle.* Because many countries' legal limits for driving are well below the level of alcohol necessary to be considered drunk or intoxicated, this issue is not addressed further in this case study. In other contexts, what is prohibited under the rubric of intoxication or drunkenness is often expressed by focusing on associated behavior, such as lack of motor coordination or causing a nuisance.

There are many variations in the circumstances that might lead to criminalization of drunkenness, such as whether the intoxication occurs in public or private, whether any other criminal act is connected to the intoxication (e.g., assault, causing a public nuisance, or operating a vehicle, a boat, or an aircraft with BAC above the legislated limit), and, if intoxication is linked to alcoholism, whether it should be treated as a disease rather than punished as a crime. Finally, a related issue is whether criminal penalties, civil penalties, or both should be imposed on a person who contributes to or encourages the intoxication, particularly if the intoxicated person goes on to injure an innocent third party. It is these situations that are the focus of this case study.

INTOXICATION AND CRIMINALITY

Intoxication as a Defense

Intoxication may be raised as a defense to certain criminal charges, on the grounds that a sufficiently high degree of alcohol-related impairment can affect the state of mind, known as *mens rea*, that is required to commit many criminal offenses. This issue raises some rather technical questions of mental capacity and intent, and its object is not to control drunkenness per se, but rather to take into account the physiological effect of intoxication on one's motivation and behavior. Put simply, the concern is to ensure that the accused does not indirectly benefit from becoming drunk voluntarily and subsequently attempting to use the fact of his or her intoxication to argue that the requisite intent to commit a crime did not exist, thus excusing acts that would have been criminal had he or she been sober. When permitted, the

* For a table listing maximum BAC limits for driving in different countries, see http://www.icap.org/Table/BACLimitsWorldwide

defense of intoxication prevents a person from being punished for having a criminal intent that he or she did not, in fact, possess.

Public Drunkenness

The short title of an early 17th-century English statute reflects the attitude toward drunkenness at the time: *An Act for Repressing the Odious and Loathsome Sin of Drunkenness* (cited in Simester & Brookbanks, 2002, p. 299). The combination of the moral disapproval of drinking that still exists in many societies and the desire to protect the public from possible antisocial aspects of public intoxication have led many jurisdictions to either punish drunkenness per se or punish drunkenness as an offense closely related to other behavior, such as the common crime of being "drunk and disorderly."

The latter combination appears to be the most widespread way in which intoxication and drunkenness are dealt with in the criminal law. In the United States, for example, most prohibitions against drunkenness include a requirement that the person also be disorderly or in some other manner commit an objectionable act, in addition to simply being drunk. A typical statute is that found in the state of Michigan, which defines a "disorderly person" as, *inter alia,* "A person who is intoxicated in a public place *and* who is either endangering directly the safety of another person or of property or is acting in a manner that causes a public disturbance" (see Sec. 750.167(1e) in Legislative Council, State of Michigan, 2009, italics added). The Republic of Ireland criminalizes both public intoxication and the potential for disorderly conduct, by providing that "[i]t shall be an offence for any person to be present in any public place while intoxicated to such an extent as would give rise to a reasonable apprehension that he might endanger himself or any other person in his vicinity" (see Sec. 4(1) in Office of the Attorney General, 1994).* A formulation that focuses on associated acts rather than potential danger is found in the state of Georgia, where a person can be convicted for public drunkenness only when that condition "is made manifest by boisterousness, by indecent

* In the United States, Texas has a similar statute that makes public drunkenness a Class C misdemeanor. Texas tourism officials expressed concern that a highly publicized crackdown on drunkenness in 2006 might hurt the state's popularity as a tourist destination ("Texas Tourism Officials," 2006).

condition or act, or by vulgar, profane, loud, or unbecoming language" (see Title 16, Sec. 16-11-41(a), in Georgia General Assembly, n.d.).*

Some jurisdictions do punish the mere fact of being intoxicated. For example, in the state of Indiana, "It is a Class B misdemeanor for a person to be in a public place or a place of public resort in a state of intoxication caused by the person's use of alcohol or a controlled substance" (see IC 7.1-5-1-3 in Indiana Legislative Services Agency, 2007). More common today, however, is provision that a person intoxicated in public can be detained by the authorities but without being deemed to have committed a criminal offense. The state of Montana, for example, specifically excludes public intoxication per se from the criminal law: "A person who appears to be intoxicated in public does not commit a criminal offense solely by reason of being in an intoxicated condition but may be detained by a peace officer for the person's own protection. … [A] peace officer may detain a person who appears to be intoxicated until the person is no longer creating a risk to self or others" (see Sec. 53-24-107(1) and (2) in Montana Legislative Services, 2009). France appears to adopt a similar stance, insofar as it permits the police to detain any person in a state of public intoxication until that person has "recovered his senses";† no criminal liability attaches (see Art. L3341-1 in Légifrance, 2010). South Australia also provides for temporary detention of any person "who is in a public place [and who] is under the influence of a drug or alcohol … and … that by reason of that fact the person is unable to take proper care of himself" (see Sec. 7(1) in Government of South Australia, Attorney-General's Department, 1984).

These laws to punish or control public drunkenness are based not only on society's determination of what constitutes acceptable behavior, but on subjective definitions of that behavior. As noted earlier, the concept of public drunkenness depends on the perception of the arresting or detaining officer (and subsequently a judge or jury), who is

* Georgia courts have held that it is not a crime to be intoxicated without manifesting one of the elements mentioned in the statute (see *Ferguson v. City of Doraville,* 1988).

† The original text in French is as follows, "Une personne trouvée en état d'ivresse dans les rues, chemins, places, cafés, cabarets ou autres lieux publics, est, par mesure de police, conduite à ses frais au poste le plus voisin ou dans une chambre de sûreté, pour y être retenue jusqu'à ce qu'elle ait recouvré la raison" (see Art. L3341-1 in Légifrance, 2010).

supposed to determine whether a person is, for example, "boisterous," "profane," "causing a nuisance," "unable to care for himself," or "posing a danger to himself or others." Unlike the BAC-focused approach taken in certain alcohol-impaired driving statutes, this approach implicitly recognizes that different people metabolize and react to alcohol differently, and it is the manifestations of intoxication that are generally deemed to be antisocial or criminal.* The New South Wales Intoxicated Persons Act 1979 (since repealed), for example, defined an intoxicated person simply as "a person who appears to be seriously affected by alcohol or another drug or a combination of drugs" (see Sec. 3 in Australasian Legal Information Institute, 2005). This air of subjectivity makes generalizations about legally defining intoxication almost impossible.

Even though such definitions are relatively vague, constitutional challenges to this vagueness have not been successful. For example, a California statute defines disorderly conduct as including, *inter alia,* any person "who is found in any public place under the influence of intoxicating liquor or any drug, in such a condition that s/he is unable to exercise care for his or her own safety or the safety of others" (see Sec. 647 (f) in Legislative Council, State of California, n.d). This language was upheld as constitutionally sufficient by the U.S. Court of Appeals for the Ninth Circuit, which found that "the requirement of reasonable certainty in statutes affecting individuals does not preclude the use of ordinary terms to express ideas which find adequate interpretation in common usage and understanding" (*Budd v. Madigan,* 1969, p. 1035).

Finally, a somewhat different but related category is the protection of minors from the effects of alcohol, which could be achieved by criminalizing both the intoxication of the minor and the person who provided the alcohol. In this situation, the concern is not so much with alcohol or even intoxication, but with protecting young people under the minimum drinking age, as defined by a given jurisdiction, from

* An Australian report identified the following factors as influencing the effect of a drug (including alcohol) on an individual: quantity of drug taken; method of drug use; a person's physical characteristics, psychological state, and previous experience with drugs; genetic factors; and whether other drugs are also used. It concluded, "This means that it is impossible to accurately predict the impact of drugs and alcohol upon individuals" (Tasmania Law Reform Institute, 2005, paras. 2.4.2–2.4.3).

alcohol's potentially harmful effects, in a manner similar to other laws with the purpose of restricting minors from engaging in behavior that is legal for adults. There is generally no distinction drawn in alcohol-specific laws between underage drinking (irrespective of quantity) and underage intoxication.* However, an adult who facilitates a minor's intoxication might also be charged with the more general criminal offense of contributing to the delinquency of a minor.

Private Intoxication

What all of these laws have in common is that, except in the case of underage youth, they punish only *public* intoxication. *Private* intoxication is commonly addressed, if it is addressed at all, as a public health issue, either as a symptom of alcoholism or as part of broader government campaigns to ensure that the public does not abuse potentially harmful substances or to promote healthier lifestyles. In France, for example, although the state is committed to treating and preventing alcoholism, this is to be accomplished through publicity, education, and treatment in medical facilities, not through the criminalization of alcoholism itself (see Art. L3311-1–L3311-4 in Légifrance, 2010).

Private intoxication also falls within the zone of individual private choice recognized under international human rights law, although international law does permit rights to be restricted, when necessary, on grounds such as the protection of public health or the rights of others.† Although one scholar has observed that "it is not clear whether there are any instances of private conduct which are proscribable *just* because they are offensive to public morality" (Janis, Kay, & Bradley, 2008, p. 428, italics in original), an analogy with the prohibition of the use of certain drugs, even in private, suggests that protection of an individual's health might entitle the government to punish private drunkenness. However, any such limitation on privacy rights must not be arbitrary or unreasonable; government does not enjoy unlimited

* For a table listing minimum age limits to drink and purchase alcohol in different countries, see http://www.icap.org/Table/MinimumAgeLimitsWorldwide

† A specific right to privacy is protected in, *inter alia,* the International Covenant on Civil and Political Rights (see Art. 17 in United Nations General Assembly, 1966), the European Convention for the Protection of Human Rights and Fundamental Freedoms (see Art. 8 in Council of Europe, 1950), and the American Convention on Human Rights (see Art. 11 in Inter-American Commission on Human Rights, 1969).

discretion to limit internationally recognized rights.* In any event, punishment of private intoxication is not common, although abolitionist jurisdictions obviously may punish the possession, sale, or use of any quantity of alcohol.

Civil Liability for Abetting Drunkenness

One is not normally under a legal duty to care for others, and civil liability attaches under the common law only when one causes harm to an innocent party deliberately or through negligence or recklessness. Historically, this had in the past led courts to reject imposing liability on the service of alcohol to a person who subsequently harms an innocent party due to being intoxicated, as the "proximate cause" of the intoxication is consuming (too many) drinks, not the serving of the drinks. In more modern times, however, many jurisdictions have enacted *dram shop laws* (so named because gin was sold in 18th-century England by the spoonful, or dram) that impose civil liability on pub or bar owners serving alcohol to patrons who (generally) are either drunk or becoming drunk. Similar laws may extend liability to social (i.e., private) hosts, as well, as it has been done, for example, in a number of U.S. states that hold adults criminally and civilly liable when they provide alcohol to underage young people in their own home.†

Because many intoxicated drivers (most of the cases seem to arise in the context of motor vehicle crashes) have few assets with which to compensate their victims, a number of jurisdictions have decided to shift the financial burden that otherwise would fall on the victim to those who can bear it more easily—the pub, the bar, or the restaurant. The determination as to whether to impose liability is thus essentially one of allocating costs to spread financial losses more broadly throughout the society: "[E]ither alcohol servers absorb the cost of increased insurance premiums, or third party victims are forced to forego recovery of compensation" (Votava, 2001, p. 605).

---

* For example, article 8.2 of the European Convention for the Protection of Human Rights and Fundamental Freedoms requires that limitations on private life be "necessary in a democratic society in the interests of national security, public safety or the economic well-being of the country, for the prevention of disorder or crime, for the protection of health or morals, or for the protection of the rights and freedoms of others" (Council of Europe, 1950, Art. 8.2).

† For an overview of this topic, see the Alcohol Policy Information System at http://alcoholpolicy.niaaa.nih.gov/

Another common argument in favor of imposing liability is that it "can help prevent problems by shaping the environment in which alcohol is sold" (Marin Institute, n.d., para. 4), by encouraging bar owners to act more responsibly.* Of course, there may be significant problems in determining just what degree of care should be exercised, particularly if drinks are ordered by one person for others or when a patron's degree of intoxication may not be readily observable. Another problem is how to apportion blame in cases of "bar-hopping," when drinking is spread over several different establishments: Should the first server be liable for contributing to the eventual drunkenness, even if the patron was relatively sober at the time? Whether dram shop laws do, in fact, encourage more responsible serving is difficult to determine, particularly because the scope of liability varies so much from jurisdiction to jurisdiction.

In the United States, a majority of the 50 states have adopted some form of dram shop statute, although the extent of liability imposed on servers differs considerably (Votava, 2001). Most states impose liability when alcohol is served to already intoxicated patrons or underage young people, with variations as to whether a plaintiff must prove that a server actually knew or only should have known that the patron was intoxicated or under the legal drinking age. Most states also limit the amount of damages that can be obtained from the serving establishment.

CONCLUSION

Every country adopts laws based on its own concept of morality, and it is obvious that there is a great range of views on alcohol, from total prohibition to widespread tolerance of alcohol consumption and even drunkenness. International human rights law permits the limitation of many rights on the ground of public morals—as well as public health and safety—although such limitations must be reasonable and proportional. Even within countries, as is the case in the United States under the provisions of the 21st Amendment to the Constitution, there may be no uniformity in the way in which different regions or cities regulate the importation, distribution, and consumption of alcohol.

---

* For example, the Marin Institute (n.d.) reported on a 2005 case in the state of New Jersey, in which the family of a girl paralyzed in an automobile accident caused by a drunk driver was awarded $135 million, split equally between the driver and the corporate owner of the beer concession at the New York Giants football stadium, where the alcohol was served.

Laws are an essential adjunct to the way in which a society enforces its moral judgments, but there are no fundamental legal principles that govern the way in which the law is used with respect to alcohol intoxication. Apart from the prohibition against unreasonable discrimination (e.g., applying different rules to different ethnic groups or distinguishing between men and women), public authorities are free to use legal mandates to reflect their own views of whether criminalization, protective detention, treatment, or laissez-faire policies are best suited to deal with a given case.

The concept of intoxication or drunkenness itself is ill defined, depending on the actions of the drinker rather than any scientific determination as to how much alcohol is "too much." Except where alcohol is banned or where specific laws address minors, it is generally only public, not private, intoxication that is legally prohibited. Laws cannot totally substitute for morality nor perfectly control human behavior—murder has been illegal since time immemorial, for example, although it continues to be committed—and the most effective means of minimizing the negative outcomes of intoxication are more likely to be through education, changing attitudes, and social pressure to drink responsibly. For adults, regulating intoxication per se through law, whether criminal or civil, will rarely be the most powerful tool available, although criminal sanctions for public drunkenness may have value as a short-term response to particular situations and prohibiting operation of vehicles, boats, or aircraft while intoxicated has shown to be effective in reducing such conduct.

Like legal definitions, clinical definitions of what it means to be intoxicated are linked to displays of impairment rather than specific BAC measures or the amount of alcohol consumed.

Clinical Definitions of Intoxication

Acute alcohol intoxication is a diagnostic entity in the two principal international systems of diagnosis and classification: the International Classification of Diseases, currently in its 10th revision (ICD–10; World Health Organization, 1992), and the *Diagnostic and Statistical Manual of Mental Disorders* (4th ed., text revision [*DSM–IV–TR*]) of the American

Psychiatric Association (2000). The definitions of acute alcohol intoxication in these two systems are conceptually similar: It is defined in both as a short-term state that occurs after drinking and has features compatible with the known physiological effects of alcohol, including euphoria, disinhibition, talkativeness, slurred speech, and, at higher doses, lack of coordination, unsteady gait, involuntary eye movement (nystagmus), memory impairment, lack of attention, stupor, and coma. Implicit in the diagnosis is that other causes of these states have been excluded. The state of intoxication is time limited: When alcohol is no longer present, having been eliminated from the body, the person essentially returns to the state that existed prior to drinking. There are no continuing effects (for a healthy adult), unless specific complications have ensued, such as hypoxia or head trauma—or unless the acute intoxication is regularly repeated (chronic). It should be noted that the actual blood, breath, or tissue alcohol concentration does not enter into consideration for the diagnosis; rather, the diagnosis is made on clinical criteria and on evidence that alcohol has been consumed.

Both ICD–10 and *DSM–IV–TR* systems state that the condition follows the consumption of alcohol to the extent that there are resultant disturbances in consciousness, cognition, perception, affect, behavior, or other psychophysiological functions and responses, which are summarized in *DSM–IV–TR* as maladaptive behavioral or psychological changes, illustrated by such outcomes as inappropriate sexual or aggressive behavior, mood lability, impaired judgment, or impaired social and occupational functions. The disturbances are directly related to the acute pharmacological effects of alcohol. In ICD–10, alcohol intoxication is synonymous with "acute drunkenness in alcoholism," although alcoholism itself is not a diagnostic term in ICD–10, and "drunkenness" is not otherwise specified. The principal international diagnostic systems, therefore, make no differentiation between acute intoxication and drunkenness. What do the clinical symptoms of intoxication mean, however, and how are they experienced by the drinker?

"Real-Life" Experience of Intoxication

The experience of intoxication begins as an extension of the usual and expected effects of alcohol. The cerebral cortex of the brain is affected by alcohol after an individual consumes one or two 10-g drinks within 1 hour. A person in normal health might experience a sense of relaxation, well-being, and, perhaps, a loss of inhibition, which may be manifest in talkativeness and euphoria, as well as a sensation of light-headedness, although these behavioral manifestations are largely culture-specific. There is usually no loss of coordination at this stage, although perception and processing of visual information (i.e., total response and motor response time to optical stimuli and decision time about sequential optical stimuli) can become impaired (Breitmeier, Seeland-Schulze, Hecker, & Schneider, 2007).

Indeed, the literature suggests that cognitive processes are affected before—that is, at a lower BAC than—impairment of motor processes or motor function. Cognitive processes are the basic mental abilities we use to think, study, and learn, including our ability to analyze sounds and images, recall information from memory, make associations among different pieces of information, and maintain concentration on particular tasks. Motor or psychomotor function is the muscular activity and movement directly resulting from mental processes. Motor skills are actions that involve the movement of muscles in the body. They are divided into two groups: gross motor skills, which include the larger movements of arms, legs, feet, or the entire body; and fine motor skills, which are small movements of the hands, wrists, fingers, feet, toes, lips, and tongue. Alcohol interferes with the neuronal messages from the brain to muscles, resulting in impaired motor function and, hence, skills. Table 2.1 summarizes the typical physiological effects (including cognitive and motor impairments) that can be observed within a certain BAC range for a novice drinker; these effects, however, are also influenced by age and gender, as well as genetic, subjective, and task factors (further discussed later). Consequently, the effect and impairment of an individual may be unpredictable, with BAC and the number of drinks consumed serving as poor measures of intoxication and potential outcomes. Observable cognitive and motor impairment following alcohol consumption generally only occurs at a BAC of 0.3 mg/ml or above, although it can be measured at 0.2 mg/ml for some alcohol effects (Moskowitz, Burns, Fiorentino, Smiley, & Zador, 2000; Moskowitz & Fiorentino, 2000).

When alcohol consumption ceases, the BAC decreases. An individual with a steadily declining BAC reaches a state of relative dysphoria and physical discomfort, namely, a *hangover*. This is generally accompanied by low energy, as restorative (REM) sleep is inhibited by alcohol intoxication.

As BAC declines, the person could experience nausea (a response to autonomic hyperactivity affecting the gut), vomiting, headache, aching limbs, sweating, and gooseflesh. Alcohol-induced diuresis (the increased formation of urine by the kidneys) causes dehydration, which contributes to the headache and aching limbs, unless an appropriate nonalcoholic fluid intake is maintained. Although the hangover can continue even when the BAC has declined to zero, alcohol intoxication is a time-limited state.

Blackouts

As noted in Table 2.1, at higher doses, alcohol can interfere with the ability to form new memories. A common consequence of clinically significant alcohol intoxication is partial (i.e., fragmentary) or complete (i.e., en bloc) memory loss, commonly known as a *blackout* (complete anterograde amnesia), which is a period of memory loss for events that transpired while an individual was intoxicated. Unlike alcohol-induced sleep or alcohol-induced unconsciousness, blackouts do not involve a loss of consciousness, just a loss of memory. An individual experiencing a fragmentary blackout may gradually recollect events and recover memory for the lost period.

The typical blackout lasts approximately 2 to 6 hours, generally corresponding to the drinker's peak BAC. As BAC rises, the likelihood of a blackout increases (Perry et al., 2006), but BAC alone does not predict a blackout. Studies in which respondents reporting blackouts have consumed alcohol in controlled conditions show that a blackout is experienced in approximately one third of episodes of induced intoxication (e.g., O'Mahony, 2004). Importantly, the rate at which alcohol is consumed and the rate at which the BAC rises have been linked to the likelihood of a blackout (Ryback, 1970).

Possible mechanisms for a blackout include alcohol-induced hypoglycemia or a low blood glucose level. Mechanisms underlying alcohol-induced memory impairments involve disruptions of activity in the hippocampus, a brain region that plays a central role in the formation of new autobiographical memories (White, 2003). Thus, brain and head injury and consequent concussion may also be mechanisms for some but not all events, as is brain damage from recurrent clinically significant alcohol intoxication.

TABLE 2.1

Physiological Effects and Impairment That May Be Observed Within a Certain Blood Alcohol Concentration Range for a Novice Drinker

BAC Range (in mg/ml)	Effects and Possible Impairment
0.3–0.4	Possible impairment of the drinker's: • Ability to detect acoustic signals and process visual information (Mann, Cho-Young, & Vogel-Sprott, 1984; Moskowitz & Murray, 1976; Schneider & Carpenter, 1969). • Divided-attention performance (Moskowitz & Sharma, 1974; Palva, Linnoila, Routledge, & Seppälä, 1982). • Eye–hand performance (Price & Flax, 1982).
0.5–0.8	• The cerebral cortex and forebrain are affected by alcohol. • The relaxed feeling can lead to a loss of alertness, and a further loss of inhibition, excessive talkativeness, and self-confidence. • There could be a decline in judgment, reasoning, and psychomotor skills (in many countries, the maximum BAC limit to drive is set within this range). For example, as the BAC approaches 0.8 mg/ml, the following functions may become impaired: • Information processing (Hernández, Vogel-Sprott, Huchín-Ramirez, & Aké-Estrada, 2006; Moskowitz & Burns, 1971; Moskowitz & DePry, 1968; Moskowitz & Murray, 1976; Moskowitz & Roth, 1971). • Perception of movement for low speeds (MacArthur & Sekuler, 1982). • Visual tracking ability (Linnoila, Erwin, & Cleveland, 1978; Linnoila, Erwin, & Ramm, 1980). • Sensorimotor coordination; that is, hand–eye coordination, motor speed, and motor function (Cherry et al., 1983). • Capacity for free recall, which improves on cuing (Birnbaum, Parker, Hartley, & Noble, 1978). • Attention performance (Burns & Moskowitz, 1980), with an increased number of mistakes in single-reaction and extended exercises and an increased response time (Bartl, Lager, & Domesle, 1996; Gustafson, 1986; Landauer & Howat, 1983; Linnoila et al., 1978; Linnoila et al., 1980).
0.9–1.4	• Cerebral cortex, forebrain, and cerebellum are affected by alcohol. • Speech can be slurred. • Balance and coordination are impaired (Perham, Moore, Shepherd, & Cusens, 2007), with visible body sway (Nieschalk et al., 1999). • Auditory and visual attention, including color perception (Grütters, Reichelt, Ritz-Timme, Thome, & Kaatsch, 2003; Wallgren & Barry, 1970), are impaired.

TABLE 2.1 (CONTINUED)

Physiological Effects and Impairment That May Be Observed Within a Certain Blood Alcohol Concentration Range for a Novice Drinker

BAC Range (in mg/ml)	Effects and Possible Impairment
	• Reaction time and reflexes are slowed (Wallgren & Barry, 1970), behavior might become exaggerated and unstable. • Nausea and vomiting can occur.
1.5–2.0	• In addition to experiencing significant impairment in simple reaction times (Wallgren & Barry, 1970), an individual can feel confused, disoriented, dazed, sedated, and sleepy. The drinker's eyes might appear to be "glazed over" (Perham et al., 2007). • The drinker might have difficulty moving (Perham et al., 2007). • Behavior can vary from quiet sedation to, in some specific cases and under unique circumstances, abusive and aggressive behavior. • Temporary losses of consciousness and, hence, a partial or total memory loss (blackouts) are typical in this BAC range.
2.1–2.5	• The cerebral cortex, forebrain, cerebellum, and brain stem are affected by alcohol. • An individual could have a staggering gait, "glazed" eyes, and slurred speech (Perham et al., 2007).
2.6–3.0 and above	• The entire brain is affected by alcohol, including the central breathing or respiratory center, located in the medulla oblongata, the lower part of the brain stem. • The person is typically unconscious or even comatose, which is a deep and prolonged unconsciousness. • The nerves that control involuntary actions such as breathing and the gag reflex (which prevents choking) are depressed or paralyzed. • Bladder control may be impaired. • The risk of death increases progressively as the BAC rises beyond 3.0 mg/ml. Death may occur when the BAC is 4.0 mg/ml or greater.

HOW AND WHY DO YOU GET INTOXICATED?

Water-soluble alcohol readily and rapidly crosses biological membranes, such as the blood–brain barrier, and passes into the brain. The extent of its distribution into the brain regions broadly correlates with the BAC, where the actual brain alcohol concentration also approximates the BAC. Because brain alcohol concentrations are difficult to measure directly, however, the effects of alcohol on the brain are calculated indirectly by observing the cognitive and psychomotor impairments that typically arise at various levels of BAC.

Alcohol exerts both general and specific dose-dependent effects on the brain. Once in the brain, alcohol affects the composition and microstructure of biological membranes, including that of brain nerve cells or neurons that generate and conduct nerve electrical messages or signals. The brain essentially contains circuits of interconnected neurons that pass or transmit information controlling individual actions and behavior. Neurotransmitters (chemical messengers) diffuse out of the neuron, cross the gap (or synapse) between the neurons, and bind to receptors on the next neuron's cell membrane, causing its ion channels to open, thus transmitting the signal. Alcohol alters the configuration of fatty acid chains in neuronal membranes (Hunt, 1985; Tabakoff, Hoffman, Valverius, Nhamburo, & Saito, 1988); this, in turn, can alter the chemical communication or signaling between neurons.

Alcohol's Effect on Neurotransmitters

The neurotransmitters primarily affected by alcohol are gamma-aminobutyric acid (GABA), adenosine, glutamate, dopamine, serotonin, and opioid peptides. These neurotransmitters fall into three categories: excitatory, which activate the postsynaptic cell; inhibitory, which depress the activity of the postsynaptic cell; and neuromodulators, which modify the postsynaptic cell's response to other neurotransmitters. Under normal conditions, a balance exists between excitatory and inhibitory neurotransmission in the brain. Acute or short-term exposure to alcohol tilts this balance toward inhibition by both increasing the function of inhibitory neurotransmitters and decreasing the function of excitatory neurotransmitters.

Simply put, alcohol is largely a depressant, which means that it slows the activity and information processing in the central nervous system, increasing the time needed to react, impairing decision making, and reducing motor control. Interestingly, these depressive effects may also explain the stimulatory effects of alcohol. The brain contains inhibitory centers (cells and circuits) that ordinarily moderate a person's behavior. Alcohol depresses the activity of these centers. As there are six different neurotransmitters affected by alcohol, a person's behavior is influenced by a complex interaction of the depressive effects of alcohol on these different inhibitory and excitatory neurotransmitters, located in different areas of the brain. As BAC increases, more areas of the brain—and, accordingly, more neurotransmitters—become affected by alcohol.

Inhibitory and Excitatory Processes

Alcohol's immediate effect is to increase the inhibition caused by the GABA, the main inhibitory neurotransmitter in the brain (which acts through a receptor subtype $GABA_A$) to produce anti-anxiolytic and sedating effects. Although GABA-mediated inhibition occurs in all brain regions, alcohol increases the ability of GABA to open the chloride ion channel for only some sorts of $GABA_A$ receptors. When the BAC is over 2.5 mg/ml, alcohol opens the chloride ion channel independently of GABA, allowing an excessive chloride influx that can result in paralysis of the neurons responsible for respiration, leading to asphyxiation. Alcohol also inhibits the degradation of GABA, thereby increasing its concentration as well as function. Thus, the anti-anxiolytic sedating effects of alcohol are primarily mediated by increasing the concentration and function of GABA. In addition, alcohol increases the activity of adenosine, another inhibitory neurotransmitter, causing sedation.*

Sedation is also caused by alcohol decreasing the activity or function of glutamate, the main excitatory neurotransmitter at the N-methyl-D-aspartate (NMDA) glutamate receptor, which sits in the cell membrane and allows the influx of calcium ions into the cell to excite it. Alcohol blocks glutamate from binding to the receptor and closes the calcium ion channel, thus decreasing primary excitatory signaling throughout the brain. In turn, the altered excitatory signaling reduces the NMDA-mediated release of other neurotransmitters such as dopamine, norepinephrine, and acetylcholine. Glutamate activity is related to cognition, learning, and memory—activities that therefore become impaired by alcohol. The decreased activity of glutamate is also associated with alcohol-induced blackouts, described earlier.

---

* Conversely, caffeine decreases the activity of adenosine, causing stimulation.

Other Neurotransmitters

Unlike GABA and glutamate, dopamine and serotonin can either stimulate or inhibit signals, depending on the area of the brain in which they are situated.

Dopamine

Alcohol increases the synthesis and release of dopamine in the nucleus accumbens (a collection of neurons thought to play an important role in pleasure, reward, laughter, addiction, fear, and the placebo effect), situated in the forebrain, and in the ventral tegmental area (VTA; linked to, e.g., the brain's reward system), situated in the midbrain. Alcohol hence increases the information relay from the VTA to the nucleus accumbens by the dopaminergic neurons, which increases the synthesis and release of dopamine in the core of the nucleus accumbens. Dopamine itself does not excite or inhibit its target neurons but acts by altering the sensitivity of its target neurons to other neurotransmitters, particularly glutamate, as well as altering the release of other neurotransmitters. Apart from motivation and reward, and an ability to experience pleasure and pain, dopamine is involved in behavior, emotion, and mood, as well as in cognition and motor skills.

Serotonin

Serotonin is also involved in the regulation of behavior, emotion, and mood, including both euphoria and depression, as well as arousal, sleep, and appetite and consumption behaviors. Used by numerous neurons situated throughout the brain, alcohol increases the release of serotonin from the different serotonin receptor subtypes, each of which has its own specific influence on behavior. Serotonin may alter the rate at which its target neurons produce electrical signals or may alter the release of other transmitters such as GABA and dopamine by the cell. Indeed, alcohol does not only affect these neurotransmitters individually but also influences their interaction. For example, serotonin can interact with neurons that synthesize and release GABA. If alcohol is present, the alcohol-influenced serotonin can affect the actions of GABA neurons in areas involving behavior such as the hippocampus (Kawa, 1994), where cognitive decisions are made and may contribute to alcohol-induced memory loss and impaired judgment. Similarly, alcohol-influenced serotonin stimulates dopamine synthesis and release in the VTA (Brodie, Trifunovic, & Shefner, 1995; Campbell, Kohl, & McBride, 1996) and, hence, nucleus accumbens, thus also being involved in pleasure, motivation, and reward reactions.

Opioids

Opioid peptide neurotransmitters, referred to as *neuromodulators,* include endorphin and enkephalin. They are involved in the management of pain by promoting analgesia, the regulation of appetite and consumption behaviors, and the reinforcement of continued alcohol consumption via modulating the effects of other neurotransmitters (Froehlich, 1997). There is a genetic variation in the effects of alcohol on the synthesis and release of opioids—for example, there is greater stimulation and release of beta-endorphins by alcohol in individuals with a family history of alcohol dependence than in individuals with no such family history (e.g., Froehlich, 1997; Froehlich & Li, 1994).

Hormones

Furthermore, the interactions of alcohol with the multiple neurotransmitter and second messenger systems are also affected by hormones, some of which differ between male and female brains. Although alcohol's actions are not mediated primarily by circulating hormones, it stimulates the synthesis and release of hormones produced by the adrenal gland, part of hypothalamic pituitary axis. The hormones include those of the adrenal cortex such as cortisol (Aguirre, del Arbol, Rico, Raya, & Ruiz-Requena, 1995; Schuckit, Gold, & Risch, 1987; Veldman & Meinders, 1996; Walter & Noth, 1984) and those of the adrenal medulla such as adrenaline (A) and noradrenaline (NA).

Cortisol

Cortisol is a component of the body's stress response system. The release of cortisol can focus alertness and attention and increase blood pressure; cortisol can also suppress bone growth, digestion, reproduction, and wound repair. A high BAC may be interpreted by the body and brain as "stress," as alcohol directly affects the chemicals that signal the adrenal glands to synthesize and release cortisol. An increased concentration of cortisol can induce depression (Brown & Suppes, 1998), impair cognitive functioning (de Quervain, Roozendaal, Nitsch, McGaugh, & Hock, 2000; Keenan et al., 1996; Newcomer et al., 1999; Wolkowitz et al., 1990), and alter sleep patterns all of which are associated with, and potentially additive to, the effects of alcohol on neurotransmitters.

Testosterone

Synthesis and release of the steroid or sex hormone, testosterone, can be either stimulated or inhibited by alcohol in the adrenal cortex or peripherally in both men (in testes) and women (in ovaries), depending on the amount and pattern of alcohol consumed and the drinker's individual characteristics (Sarkola & Eriksson, 2003; Sierksma et al., 2004). The blood testosterone concentration after drinking is the result of the net effect of an inhibited liver metabolism of testosterone and an inhibited synthesis of testosterone in the gonads (testes in men and ovaries in women). It would, therefore, depend on different hormonal conditions as well as different amounts and patterns of alcohol consumption—so, for example, the inhibited synthesis of testosterone may predominate after large amounts of alcohol are consumed over a short period of time, and also when, in the late descending phase of alcohol elimination, all the alcohol consumed has been completely metabolized.

Other Hormones

In addition, alcohol inhibits the release of antidiuretic hormone (ADH), or arginine vasopressin, from the posterior pituitary gland. The decreased concentration of ADH prevents the kidneys from reabsorbing water, thus promoting water loss, which increases the rate of urine formation. The concentration of blood electrolytes correspondingly increases, resulting in dehydration.

The Effects of Alcohol on the Developing Brain

It was initially thought that brain development was essentially completed by adolescence, but it is now accepted that the brain continues to develop into adulthood. The prefrontal cortex, limbic brain regions such as the hippocampus, white matter myelin, and reward circuits all undergo active development during adolescence (Chambers, Taylor, & Potenza, 2003; Spear, 2000). Consequently, these structures and their functions of cognitive, behavioral, and emotional regulation can be particularly vulnerable to the adverse effects of alcohol. Alternatively, it has been argued that deficits or developmental delays in these structures and their functions may predispose adolescents to accelerated alcohol consumption patterns and, potentially, alcohol dependence (Clark, Thatcher, & Tapert, 2008). For example, the brains of adolescents who habitually consume large amounts of alcohol have smaller prefrontal white matter volumes compared to those of control adolescents (De Bellis et al., 2005; Medina et al., 2008), which correlates with impaired cognitive function; the hippocampus volume, which influences both inhibitory and excitatory mechanisms, is similarly smaller in the former group (De Bellis et al., 2000). Interestingly, there appear to be gender differences in the effects of alcohol on the developing brain (Medina et al., 2008), which may reflect gender differences in the rate and timing of brain development in adolescence: The brains of females may be more sensitive to the adverse, or neurotoxic, effects of alcohol (Hommer, Momenan, Kaiser, & Rawlings, 2001; Schweinsburg et al., 2003). The mechanism(s) by which alcohol affects brain development are, however, yet to be fully explained. Although recent research suggests that heavy alcohol consumption during adolescence and early adulthood is associated with poor cognitive function, including impaired learning and memory formation and weakened attention and visuospatial skills, research about the effects of any alcohol on the developing adolescent brain has not yet produced definitive results (Clark et al., 2008).

Other Factors Influencing Intoxication

In contrast to many other substances, alcohol is intoxicating only in large gram amounts. There is a measurable and relatively dose-dependent relationship between the amount of alcohol consumed (as a number of standard drinks) and BAC. The effects of alcohol on motor and cognitive functioning impairment, however, are not necessarily predictable from the dose and BAC, as discussed earlier. Cognitive and (psycho)motor effects are often observed for a BAC *range* rather than specific BAC levels (as demonstrated by Table 2.1). The effects of alcohol are modified by many biological factors. Indeed, the number of drinks consumed is a poor measure of intoxication because of variation in individual physiology, including height, weight, body mass index, disease, gender, and genetics, as well as concomitant food, drink, or drug intake. These additional factors modify the absorption, distribution, and elimination of alcohol and influence the resultant degree and experience of intoxication.

Food Ingestion and Beverage Type

Several factors can modify the absorption of alcohol from the stomach. Initially, the rate of absorption is rapid, but it then slows down, although the concentration of alcohol in the stomach may remain high. The presence of food delays the emptying of the contents of the stomach into the small intestine: Foods high in fat or protein significantly delay emptying and reduce maximum BAC reached. Absorption from the small intestine, however, is rapid and independent from the presence of food. Therefore, for a time, the BAC will continue to rise after consumption of the last drink. The time from the last drink to the maximum BAC usually ranges from 30 to 90 minutes, depending on whether alcohol is consumed with or without food.

Beverage type is another modifying factor of the alcohol absorption rate. For example, the higher the alcohol concentration of a drink, the faster it is absorbed from the stomach and small intestine—and so the higher the BAC. Water and fruit juices mixed with alcohol, however, slow down the absorption of alcohol from the stomach and small intestine, whereas carbonated beverages speed it up. The temperature of a drink can also make a difference: Warm alcohol is absorbed faster than cold alcohol.

Gender and Body Size Differences

A drinker's gender plays a role in the degree of intoxication: For certain cognitive and motor functions, women can be more impaired than men at the same BAC—that is, women may be more sensitive to the effects of alcohol at higher BAC levels (Bisgrove & Mills, 1983; Hommer et al., 2001; Moss, Kirisci, Gordon, & Tarter, 1994; Schweinsburg et al., 2003). Men have a higher content of body water (into which the water-soluble alcohol distributes rapidly from the blood) than women, whereas women have a higher content of body fat into which the relatively fat-insoluble alcohol distributes slowly. Alcohol distribution into and out of fat is exacerbated by a limited blood supply in fat; water-containing tissues such as muscle rapidly absorb alcohol. As the absorbed alcohol continues to circulate in the blood until it is distributed into the tissues and fluids, women record a significantly higher maximum BAC than men when a comparable concentration of alcohol is consumed. Moreover, women record a longer time for the blood alcohol to fall to baseline than men. In addition, men tend to be larger than women, and, as noted earlier, larger individuals have a higher content of body water into which alcohol distributes, as well as more metabolizing enzymes, than their smaller counterparts, recording a lower maximum BAC.

There is also a gender difference in the rate of metabolism of the ADH_7 gene and its enzyme, which breaks down alcohol in the stomach (first-pass metabolism, described earlier). The enzyme is more active in men than in women, and thus breaks down alcohol more rapidly in men (Baraona et al., 2001; Frezza et al., 1990). All this contributes to the gender difference in the maximum BAC observed.

Genetic Differences

There are at least nine forms of ADH enzymes, encoded by seven genes. Each form of the enzyme has a distinct rate of metabolism and may be located in different tissues. Different ethnic populations generally inherit different forms of these genes—and, hence, different forms of these enzymes. For example, Caucasian, Asian, and Negroid populations each have distinct forms of the ADH_2 gene and ADH_2 enzyme. Alcohol-dependent individuals, irrespective of ethnicity, do not have the form II of the ADH_2 gene, which implies that this form protects against the development of genetically or metabolically derived alcoholism (Cichoż-Lach, Celiński, & Słomka, 2008). Furthermore, for all the genes, the enzymes and their subunits have a varying affinity for alcohol and different catalytic or metabolic activity. For example, ADH_1 enzymes have a higher affinity for alcohol and are more active than the other classes in metabolizing low doses of alcohol, whereas ADH_2 and ADH_4 enzymes have a lower affinity for alcohol and are only active in metabolizing higher doses of alcohol. There is also a 20% difference in the extent of alcohol metabolism between the forms II and III of the ADH_2 enzyme. This is, therefore, the basis for variance in BAC between individuals who consume the same dose, where some individuals can be described as fast alcohol metabolizers and others as slow metabolizers.

In addition, there are three forms of the ALDH enzyme. Some Asian populations do not have the form II enzyme of the ALDH gene, which is the most active enzyme that metabolizes acetaldehyde, the primary metabolite of alcohol, to acetate (Cook et al., 2005). Therefore, many Asians cannot rapidly break down acetaldehyde, and it accumulates in the blood and tissues until it is broken down by the alternative microsomal ethanol oxidizing system (MEOS) enzyme pathway. Acetaldehyde is more toxic to the tissues than alcohol. A physical symptom of not being able to break down this primary metabolite is facial flushing, which reflects an increase in blood flow to the skin of the face, neck, and chest. Other physical symptoms include cardiovascular effects and nausea. Therefore, differences among the ADH and ALDH genes and enzymes contribute to the differences in maximum BAC observed between individuals, within and between ethnic populations.

Genetic influences on intoxication can also shape subjective responses to intoxication, sensitivity of the central nervous system to the effects of alcohol, and development of alcohol tolerance (i.e., when an individual experiences a decreased behavioral response to a given dose of alcohol after prior experience with drinking or when a greater dose of alcohol is needed to produce a given level of effect). Drinkers with a family history of alcohol dependence generally experience stronger stimulant effects when the BAC is rising, lower sedative effects when the BAC is falling, and lighter impairment than the general population, all linked to the development of alcohol dependence (Schuckit, Tsuang, Anthenelli, Tipp, & Nurnberger, 1996). Similarly, moderate-to-heavy drinkers report greater stimulant effects than lighter drinkers when the BAC is rising and lower sedative effects when the BAC is falling, which could influence the former group's habitual amount and pattern of consumption (Holdstock & de Wit, 1998, 1999; Holdstock, King, & de Wit, 2000). Sons of alcoholics tend to display less alcohol intoxication when measurements are made at least 1 hour after consuming alcohol, compared to men with no family history of alcohol dependence (Schuckit, Smith, Anderson, & Brown, 2004). Subjective intoxication ratings can be assessed through the Subjective High Assessment Scale (Schuckit & Smith, 2000) and observations of standing steadiness and body sway (Lipscomb, Carpenter, & Nathan, 1979). A low level of response to a given dose of alcohol is associated with a 40 to 60% risk of developing alcohol dependence (Schuckit, Smith, & Kalmijn, 2004); several chromosomes have been identified as contributing to the low-level response—in particular, the genes on chromosome 10 (Schuckit et al., 2005; Wilhelmsen et al., 2003).

The Rate of Alcohol Consumption and Other Pharmacokinetic Factors

The rate at which BAC rises is a pharmacokinetic factor that influences the rate of impairment. For example, rapid alcohol consumption leads to attainment of a maximum BAC in a short period of time, where the brief duration of physiological exposure may contribute to greater impairment (Mitchell, 1985; Moskowitz & Burns, 1976). The intensity of behavioral impairment after drinking, however, can be explained by both swifter rates of rise in BAC and expectations of greater impairment (Fillmore & Vogel-Sprott, 1998).

Another pharmacokinetic factor influencing the dose–response curve is whether the drinker's BAC is ascending or descending: The cognitive and motor function effects of alcohol appear to be differentially affected—the stimulatory and positive effects predominate on rising and sedative and negative effects on falling of BAC (Martin, Earleywine, Musty, Perrine, & Swift, 1993), playing a part in subjective perceptions of intoxication. The stimulatory and positive effects include elation, excitement, and talkativeness, and the sedative and negative effects include inactivity, difficulty in concentrating, sluggishness, and heavy-headedness (Earleywine, 1994). Initially, it was observed that all cognitive impairment is more pronounced when the BAC is rising (Mellanby, 1919), however, the cognitive functions of long-term verbal memory, declarative memory, and inhibitory control have since been shown to be impaired during the ascending BAC, whereas short- and long-term visual memory and visual-spatial working memory were shown only to be impaired during the descending BAC (Schweiter et al., 2005). Information processing, reaction time (or speed), and accuracy of information processing also appear to be differentially affected by rising or falling BAC (Schweizer, Jolicoeur, Vogel-Sprott, & Dixon, 2004). Reaction time improves with falling BAC for all sources of stimulus (Hernández et al., 2006), but accuracy does not and may actually worsen (Pihl, Paylan, Gentes-Hawn, & Hoaken, 2003). Interestingly, the impairment of speed and accuracy observed at a rising BAC of approximately 1.0 mg/ml is equivalent to that caused by fatigue following approximately 24 hours of sleep deprivation (Williamson & Feyer, 2000), whereas a rising BAC of approximately 0.5 mg/ml is equivalent to 17 to 19 hours of sleep deprivation. In addition, performance of motor and cognitive tasks at a BAC of 0.8 mg/ml suggests that there is impairment of both tasks during the ascending BAC, with peak impairment at peak BAC, but only a reduction in impairment for the motor task with falling BAC (Fogarty & Vogel-Sprott, 2002; Holloway, 1995). There is also acute adaptation, or tolerance (reduced impairment), at a given blood alcohol content on the falling limb of the BAC curve, which suggests that the reduction may be due to an adaptive process occurring over time.

Task Factors Influencing Alcohol Intoxication

Although cognitive impairment generally only starts to become significant at a BAC above 0.5 mg/ml (Gilg, 1996; Huckenbeck & Bonte, 2003; Kennedy, Turnage, Wilkes, & Dunlap, 1993; Mitchell, 1985; Tagawa et al., 2000), certain functions begin to show signs of weakening at a BAC of approximately 0.3 mg/ml if tasks grow in complexity and multiplicity, especially when tasks rely on perception and processing of visual information (Breitmeier et al., 2007). Studies have generally shown that, when stimuli are simple or explicit, are presented in the absence of competing demands, and involve automatic processes linked to immediate responses, the effects of alcohol consumption on performance appear limited. In contrast, when stimuli are complex and contextual, are presented when there are competing demands for processing, and involve delayed or changing response contingencies, the effects of alcohol consumption on performance become apparent. Increasing task complexity thus magnifies alcohol-related impairment (Casbon, Curtin, Lang, & Patrick, 2003; Wallgren & Barry, 1970), as does persevering with previously task-appropriate responses that are now inappropriate. The inappropriate response is essentially an automatic inclination to select and implement one response option over others, often as a result of practice or training. At particular levels, alcohol also inhibits the ability to monitor and perform more than one task simultaneously (Maylor, Rabbitt, James, & Kerr, 1992). It has been suggested that certain cognitive functions may be impaired before motor functions (Easdon & Vogel-Sprott, 2000; Hernández et al., 2006; Levine, Kramer, & Levine, 1975), and that this occurs in a selective, stepwise manner at lower BAC (Fogarty & Vogel-Sprott, 2002). Furthermore, individual perceptions of socially appropriate behavior for a given drinking context and population affect the way one reacts after drinking, whatever the accompanying task: For example, subjective feelings of intoxication in younger, compared to older, men may relate to age-related expectations (Jones & Neri, 1985).

Subjective Factors Influencing Intoxication

So, as noted earlier, an individual's cognitive expectancies about alcohol contribute to the intensity of alcohol impairment and may influence the resultant behavior: An individual tends to behave in accordance with the expected outcomes of a course of action—in this case, alcohol consumption. This has been observed in studies where some participants consumed beverage alcohol and others drank a placebo but expected it to be alcohol (e.g., Fillmore, Carscadden, & Vogel-Sprott, 1998). The expectancy and, hence, resultant impairment differs, however, according to certain environmental conditions (Fillmore & Vogel-Sprott, 1995, 1997). Consistently, maximum subjective feelings of intoxication coincide with maximum BAC and thereafter decrease in a curvilinear time course (Jones & Neri, 1985). Expectancies could contribute to individual differences in cognitive functioning under alcohol and a placebo (Fillmore & Vogel-Sprott, 1998), which implies that BAC alone as a measure of intoxication may be inadequate.

HOW CAN YOU "SOBER UP"?

As described earlier, acute alcohol intoxication is a time-limited state. Management of intoxicated individuals essentially aims to protect them against complications such as injury, self-harm, and public vulnerability. Generally, this entails ensuring that the drinker's airway is protected and that his or her pulse, blood pressure, and respiration remain within acceptable limits. Extreme BAC and intoxication may necessitate hospital admission.

Various proprietary preparations are available and advertised as sobering-up agents, including stimulants and substances designed to accelerate alcohol metabolism. Only one agent, however, consistently achieves this goal: Fructose is a naturally occurring sugar found in fruits; its metabolism facilitates faster dissociation of the alcohol dehydrogenase-NADH complex (Tygstrup, Winkler, & Lundquist, 1965), which speeds up the initial oxidation of alcohol to ALDH, acetate, and eventually carbon dioxide and water. One hundred grams of fructose can speed up alcohol metabolism by a maximum of 80% (Mascord, Smith, Starmer, & Whitfield, 1991; Sprandel, Tröger, Liebhardt, & Zöllner, 1980). Consequently, fructose is a constituent of several sobering-up agents that accelerate the rate of alcohol metabolism by up to approximately 20%. This means that, after approximately six 10-g drinks, the total period of intoxication can be reduced by 1 to 1.5 hours.

Other commonly used sobering-up agents include caffeine and guarana (which also contains caffeine). There is no scientific evidence to suggest that they improve cognitive function and motor skills, although they do appear to reduce subjective intoxication (Ferreira, de Mello, Pompéia, & de Souza-Formigoni, 2006; Ferreira, de Mello, Rossi, & Souza-Formigoni, 2004). In addition, caffeine is a mild diuretic, which can exacerbate the dehydrating effect of alcohol.

With improved knowledge of the mechanisms of alcohol on neurotransmitter pathways, there has been renewed interest in developing sobering-up agents based on reversal of the effects of alcohol on neurotransmitters. The most well-developed example is based on blocking the effects of alcohol on the GABA ionosphere complex, which mediates much of alcohol's sedating effects. Specific ionosphere receptor blockers (agonists) such as Ro15–4513 appear to reduce subjective alcohol intoxication and improve motor skills. It has not been further developed, however, due to adverse side effects. Another example is based on blocking the effects of alcohol on the opioid neurotransmitter system. The opioid antagonist naloxone reduces subjective intoxication but does not necessarily improve motor skills when administered prior to alcohol consumption (e.g., Badawy & Aliyu, 1984; Catley, Lehane, & Jones, 1981).

Hangover "Remedies"

The alcohol-induced hangover has substantial economic and health consequences. As we have discussed, hangover symptoms may include lightheadedness, nausea, impairment of concentration and memory, and coordination difficulties, all resulting from a combination of alcohol's first metabolic product, acetaldehyde, with congeners including methanol, endocrine and immune system disturbances, dehydration and electrolyte disturbances, and sleep disturbance.

Pittler, Verster, and Ernst (2005) reviewed the effectiveness of eight different agents in preventing or treating alcohol hangovers: propranolol, tropisetron, tolfenamic acid, fructose or glucose, and the dietary supplements *Borago officinalis* (borage), *Cynara scolymus* (artichoke), *Opuntia ficus-indica* (prickly pear), and a yeast-based preparation. No compelling evidence was found to suggest that any conventional or complementary intervention is effective for preventing or treating hangovers. The authors concluded that "[t]he most effective way to avoid the symptoms of an alcohol induced hangover is to practise abstinence or moderation" (Pittler et al., 2005, p. 1515). Water, however, can help to reverse the dieresis caused by alcohol and alleviate some symptoms.

CONCLUSION

The impairment that an individual drinker experiences is the result of a complex interplay of pharmacokinetic, cognitive, and cultural factors, going far beyond simple BAC measures or the number of drinks consumed. These factors can be further modified by influences in the drinking environment, physiological characteristics, and social expectations about alcohol and intoxication. The following chapters in this volume explore the social and cultural forces that influence the expression of drunkenness.

REFERENCES

Aguirre, J. C., del Arbol, J. L., Rico, J., Raya, J., & Ruiz-Requena, M. E. (1995). Effect of acute alcohol intoxication on the opioid system in humans. *Alcohol: An International Biomedical Journal, 12,* 559–562.

American Psychiatric Association. (2000). *Diagnostic and statistical manual of mental disorders* (4th ed., text revision). Washington, DC: Author.

Australasian Legal Information Institute. (2005). *New South Wales repealed acts: Intoxicated persons act 1979.* Retrieved December 20, 2009, from http://www.austlii.edu.au/au/legis/nsw/repealed_act/ipa1979233/

Badawy, A. A. B., & Aliyu, S. U. (1984). Antagonism of acute alcohol intoxication by naloxone. *Alcohol and Alcoholism, 19,* 199–201.

Baraona, E., Abittan, C. S., Dohmen, K., Moretti, M., Pozzato, G., Chayes, Z. W., et al. (2001). Gender differences in pharmacokinetics of alcohol. *Alcoholism: Clinical and Experimental Research, 25,* 502–507.

Bartl, G., Lager, F., & Domesle, L. (1996). Testleisungen bei Minderalkoholisierung [Test performance in people under minor influence of alcohol]. *Blutalkohol, 33,* 1–16.

Birnbaum, I. M., Parker, E. S., Hartley, J. T., & Noble, E. P. (1978). Alcohol and memory: Retrieval processes. *Journal of Verbal Learning and Verbal Behavior, 17,* 325–335.

Bisgrove, E., & Mills, K. C. (1983). Body sway and divided attention performance under the dose–response differences between males and females. *Alcoholism: Clinical and Experimental Research, 7,* 393–397.

Breitmeier, D., Seeland-Schulze, I., Hecker, H., & Schneider, U. (2007). The influence of blood alcohol concentrations of around 0.03% on neuropsychological functions: A double-blind, placebo-controlled investigation. *Addiction Biology, 12,* 183–189.

Brodie, M. S., Trifunovic, R. D., & Shefner, S. A. (1995). Serotonin potentiates ethanol-induced excitation of ventral tegmental area neurons in brain slices from three different rat strains. *Journal of Pharmacology and Experimental Therapeutics, 273,* 1139–1146.

Brown, E. S., & Suppes, T. (1998). Mood symptoms during corticosteroid therapy: A review. *Harvard Review of Psychiatry, 5,* 239–246.

Burns, M. M., & Moskowitz, H. A. (1980). Effects of diphenhydramine and alcohol on skills performance. *European Journal of Clinical Pharmacology, 17,* 259–266.

Budd v. Madigan, 418 F.2d 1032 (9th Cir. 1969).

Campbell, A. D., Kohl, R. R., & McBride, W. J. (1996). Serotonin-3 receptor and ethanol-stimulated somatodendritic dopamine release. *Alcohol: An International Biomedical Journal, 13,* 569–574.

Casbon, T. S., Curtin, J. J., Lang, A. R., & Patrick, C. J. (2003). Deleterious effects of alcohol intoxication: Diminished cognitive control and its behavioral consequences. *Journal of Abnormal Psychology, 112,* 476–487.

Catley, D. M., Lehane, J. R., & Jones, J. G. (1981). Failure of naloxone to reverse alcohol intoxication. *Lancet, 1*(8232), 1263.

Chambers, R. A., Taylor, J. R., & Potenza, M. N. (2003). Developmental neurocircuitry of motivation in adolescence: A critical period of addiction vulnerability. American Journal of Psychiatry, *160,* 1041–1052.

Cherry, N., Johnston, J. D., Venables, H., Waldron, H. A., Buck, L., & MacKay, C. J. (1983). The effects of toluene and alcohol on psychomotor performance. *Ergonomics, 26,* 1081–1087.

Cichoż-Lach, H., Celiński, K., & Słomka, M. (2008). Alcohol-metabolising enzyme gene polymorphisms and alcohol chronic pancreatitis among Polish individuals. *HPB, 10,* 138–143.

Clark, D. B., Thatcher, D. L., & Tapert, S. F. (2008). Alcohol, psychological dysregulation, and adolescent brain development. *Alcoholism: Clinical and Experimental Research, 32,* 375–385.

Cook, T. A., Luczak, S. E., Shea, S. H., Ehlers, C. L., Carr, L. G., & Wall, T. L. (2005). Associations of ALDH2 and ADH1B genotypes with response to alcohol in Asian Americans. *Journal of Studies on Alcohol, 66,* 196–204.

Council of Europe. (1950). *Convention for the protection of human rights and fundamental freedoms.* Retrieved December 20, 2009, from http://conventions.coe.int/Treaty/Commun/QueVoulezVous.asp?NT=005&CL= ENG

De Bellis, M. D., Clark, D. B., Beers, S. R., Soloff, P. H., Boring, A. M., Hall, J., et al. (2000). Hippocampal volume in adolescent-onset alcohol use disorders. *American Journal of Psychiatry, 157,* 737–744.

De Bellis, M. D., Narasimhan, A., Thatcher, D. L., Keshavan, M. S., Soloff, P., & Clark, D. B. (2005). Prefrontal cortex, thalamus, and cerebellar volumes in adolescents and young adults with adolescent-onset alcohol use disorders and comorbid mental disorders. *Alcoholism: Clinical and Experimental Research, 29,* 1590–1600.

de Quervain, D. J. F., Roozendaal, B., Nitsch, R. M., McGaugh, J. L., & Hock, C. (2000). Acute cortisone administration impairs retrieval of long-term declarative memory in humans. *Nature Neuroscience, 3,* 313–314.

Earleywine, M. (1994). Confirming the factor structure of the anticipated biphasic alcohol effects scale. *Alcoholism: Clinical and Experimental Research, 18,* 861–866.

Easdon, C. M., & Vogel-Sprott, M. (2000). Alcohol and behavioral control: Impaired response inhibition and flexibility in social drinkers. *Experimental and Clinical Psychopharmacology, 8,* 387–394.

Ferguson v. City of Doraville, 186 Ga. App. 430, 367 S.E.2d 551 (1988).

Ferreira, S. E., de Mello, M. T., Pompéia, S., & de Souza-Formigoni, M. L. (2006). Effects of energy drink ingestion on alcohol intoxication. *Alcoholism: Clinical and Experimental Research, 30,* 598–605.

Ferreira, S. E., de Mello, M. T., Rossi, M. V., & Souza-Formigoni, M. L. (2004). Does an energy drink modify the effects of alcohol in a maximal effort test? *Alcoholism: Clinical and Experimental Research, 28,* 1408–1412.

Fillmore, M. T., Carscadden, J. L., & Vogel-Sprott, M. (1998). Alcohol, cognitive impairment and expectancies. *Journal of Studies on Alcohol, 59,* 174–179.

Fillmore, M. T., & Vogel-Sprott, M. (1995). Expectancies about alcohol-induced motor impairment predict individual differences in responses to alcohol and placebo. *Journal of Studies on Alcohol, 56,* 90–98.

Fillmore, M. T., & Vogel-Sprott, M. (1997). Resistance to cognitive impairment under alcohol: The role of environmental consequences. *Experimental and Clinical Psychopharmacology, 5,* 251–255.

Fillmore, M. T., & Vogel-Sprott, M. (1998). Behavioral impairment under alcohol: Cognitive and pharmacokinetic factors. *Alcoholism: Clinical and Experimental Research, 22,* 1476–1482.

Fogarty, J. N., & Vogel-Sprott, M. (2002). Cognitive processes and motor skills differ in sensitivity to alcohol impairment. *Journal of Studies on Alcohol, 63,* 404–411.

Frezza, M., DiPadova, C., Pozzato, G., Terpin, M., Baraona, E., & Lieber, C. S. (1990). High blood alcohol levels in women: The role of decreased gastric alcohol dehydrogenase activity and first-pass metabolism. *New England Journal of Medicine, 322,* 95–99.

Froehlich, J. C. (1997). Physiology of opioid peptides. *Alcohol Health and Research World, 21,* 132–136.

Froehlich, J. C., & Li, T. K. (1994). Opioid involvement in alcohol drinking. *Annals of the New York Academy of Science, 739,* 156–167.

Georgia General Assembly. (n.d.). *Georgia Code - Crimes and Offenses - Title 16, Section 16-11-41(a).* Retrieved December 20, 2009, from http://law.onecle.com/georgia/16/16-11-41.html

Gilg, T. (1996). Alkohol und Verkehrssicherheit [Alcohol and road safety]. In R. Penning (Ed.), *Rechtsmedizin Systematisch* (pp. 261–290). Bremen, Germany: Uni-Med.

Government of South Australia, Attorney-General's Department. (1984). *South Australia public intoxication act 1984.* Retrieved December 20, 2009, from www.legislation.sa.gov.au

Grütters, G., Reichelt, J. A., Ritz-Timme, S., Thome, M., & Kaatsch, H. J. (2003). Beeinträchtigung der Sicherheit im Schiffsverkehr durch Alkohol Einfluss auf das Visuelle System [Impairment of safety in navigation caused by alcohol: Impact on visual function]. *Der Ophthalmologe, 100,* 391–395.

Gustafson, R. (1986). Visual attentional span as a function of a small dose of alcohol. *Perceptual and Motor Skills, 63,* 367–370.

Hernández, O., Vogel-Sprott, M., Huchín-Ramirez, T., & Aké-Estrada, F. (2006). Acute dose of alcohol affects cognitive components of reaction time to an omitted stimulus: Differences among sensory systems. *Psychopharmacology, 184,* 75–81.

Holdstock, L., & de Wit, H. (1998). Individual differences in the biphasic effects of ethanol. *Alcoholism: Clinical and Experimental Research, 22,* 1903–1911.

Holdstock, L., & de Wit, H. (1999). Ethanol impairs saccadic and smooth pursuit eye movements without producing self-reports of sedation. *Alcoholism: Clinical and Experimental Research, 23,* 664–672.

Holdstock, L., King, A. C., & de Wit, H. (2000). Subjective and objective responses to ethanol in moderate/heavy and light social drinkers. *Alcoholism: Clinical and Experimental Research, 24,* 789–794.

Holloway, F. A. (1995). Low-dose alcohol effects on human behavior and performance. *Alcohol, Drugs and Driving, 11,* 39–56.

Hommer, D., Momenan, R., Kaiser, E., & Rawlings, R. (2001). Evidence for a gender-related effect of alcoholism on brain volumes. *American Journal of Psychiatry, 158,* 198–204.

Huckenbeck, W., & Bonte, W. (2003). Alkohologie. In *Handbuch gerichtliche Medizin* (pp. 379–636). Berlin, Germany: Springer.

Hunt, W. A. (1985). *Alcohol and biological membranes.* New York: Guilford.

Indiana Legislative Services Agency. (2007). *Indiana Code (IC) 7.1-5-1-3.* Retrieved December 20, 2009, from http://www.in.gov/legislative/ic/code/title7.1/ar5/ch1.html

Inter-American Commission on Human Rights. (1969). *American convention on human rights.* Retrieved December 20, 2009, from http://www.hrcr.org/docs/American_Convention/oashr.html

Janis, M. W., Kay, R. S., & Bradley, A. W. (2008). *European human rights law: Text and material* (3rd ed.). Oxford, UK: Oxford University Press.

Jones, A. W., & Neri, A. (1985). Age-related differences in blood ethanol parameters and subjective feelings of intoxication in healthy men. *Alcohol and Alcoholism, 20,* 45–52.

Kawa, K. (1994). Distribution and functional properties of 5-HT3 receptors in rat hippocampal dentate gyrus: A patch-clamp study. *Journal of Neurophysiology, 71,* 1935–1947.

Keenan, P. A., Jacobson, M. W., Soleymani, R. M., Mayes, M. D., Stress, M. E., & Yaldoo, D. T. (1996). The effect on memory of chronic prednisone treatment in patients with systemic disease. *Neurology, 47,* 1396–1402.

Kennedy, R. S., Turnage, J. J., Wilkes, R. L., & Dunlap, W. P. (1993). Effects of graded doses of alcohol on nine computerized repeated measures tests. *Ergonomics, 36,* 1195–1222.

Kerr, W. C., Greenfield, T. K., & Midanik, L. T. (2006). How many drinks does it take you to feel drunk? Trends and predictors for subjective drunkenness. *Addiction, 101,* 1428–1437.

Landauer, A. A., & Howat, P. A. (1983). *Blood alcohol concentrations and motor vehicle accidents: A review of the evidence.* Perth: University of Western Australia.

Légifrance. (2010). *Code de la santé publique* [Code of public health]. Retrieved December 20, 2009, from http://www.legifrance.gouv.fr

Legislative Council, State of California. (n.d.). *California penal code, Section 647(f)*. Retrieved December 20, 2009, from http://www.leginfo.ca.gov/

Legislative Council, State of Michigan. (2009). *The Michigan Penal Act 328 of 1931, Section 750.167(1e)*. Retrieved December 20, 2009, from http://legislature.mi.gov/doc.aspx?mcl-750-167

Levine, J. M., Kramer, G. G., & Levine, E. N. (1975). Effects of alcohol on human performance: An integration of research findings based on an abilities classification. *Journal of Applied Psychology, 60,* 285–293.

Linnoila, M., Erwin, C. W., & Cleveland, W. P. (1978). Effects of alcohol on psychomotor performance of men and women. *Journal of Studies on Alcohol, 39,* 745–758.

Linnoila, M., Erwin, C. W., & Ramm, D. (1980). Effect of age and alcohol on psychomotor performance of men. *Journal of Studies on Alcohol, 41,* 488–495.

Lipscomb, T. R., Carpenter, J. A., & Nathan, P. E. (1979). Static ataxia: A predictor of alcoholism? *British Journal of Addiction, 74,* 289–294.

MacArthur, R. D., & Sekuler, R. (1982). Alcohol and motion perception. *Perception & Psychophysics, 31,* 502–505.

Mann, R. E., Cho-Young, J., & Vogel-Sprott, M. (1984). Retrograde enhancement by alcohol of delayed free recall performance. *Pharmacology, Biochemistry, and Behavior, 20,* 639–642.

Marin Institute. (n.d.). *Holding retailers accountable for injury and damages*. Retrieved December 20, 2009, from http://www.marininstitute.org/alcohol_policy/dramshop.htm

Martin, C. S., Earleywine, M., Musty, R. E., Perrine, M. W., & Swift, R. M. (1993). Development and validation of the biphasic alcohol effects scale. *Alcoholism: Clinical and Experimental Research, 17,* 140–146.

Mascord, D., Smith, J., Starmer, G. A., & Whitfield, J. B. (1991). Effect of fructose on alcohol metabolism and on the (lactate)/(pyruvate) ratio in man. *Alcohol and Alcoholism, 26,* 53–59.

Maylor, E. A., Rabbitt, P. M. A., James, G. H., & Kerr, S. A. (1992). Effects of alcohol, practice, and task complexity on reaction time distributions. *Quarterly Journal of Experimental Psychology, 44A,* 119–139.

Medina, K. L., McQueeny, T., Nagel, B. J., Hanson, K. L., Schweinsburg, A. D., & Tapert, S. F. (2008). Prefrontal cortex volumes in adolescents with alcohol use disorders: Unique gender effects. *Alcoholism: Clinical and Experimental Research, 32,* 386–394.

Mellanby, E. (1919). *Alcohol: Its absorption and disappearance from the blood underdifferent conditions*. London: Her Majesty's Statistical Office.

Midanik, L. T. (1999). Drunkenness, feeling the effects and 5 + measures. *Addiction, 94,* 887–897.

Mitchell, M. C. (1985). Alcohol-induced impairment of central nervous system function: Behavioral skills involved in driving. *Journal of Studies on Alcohol, 10,* 109–116.

Montana Legislative Services. (2009). *Montana code annotated 2009. Sec. 53-24-107(1) and (2)*. Retrieved December 20, 2009, from http://data.opi.mt.gov/bills/mca/53/24/53-24-107.htm

Moskowitz, H. A., & Burns, M. M. (1971). Effect of alcohol on the psychological refractory period. *Quarterly Journal of Studies on Alcohol, 32,* 782–790.

Moskowitz, H. A., & Burns, M. M. (1976). Effects of rate of drinking on human performance. *Journal of Studies on Alcohol, 37,* 598–605.

Moskowitz, H. A., Burns, M. M., Fiorentino, D., Smiley, A., & Zador, P. (2000, August). *Driver characteristics and impairment at various BACs.* Washington, DC: U.S. National Highway Traffic Safety Administration.

Moskowitz, H. A., & DePry, D. (1968). Differential effect of alcohol on auditory vigilance and divided-attention tasks. *Quarterly Journal of Studies on Alcohol, 29,* 54–63.

Moskowitz, H. A., & Fiorentino, D. (2000, April). *A review of the literature on the effects of low doses of alcohol on driving-related skills.* Washington, DC: U.S. National Highway Traffic Safety Administration.

Moskowitz, H. A., & Murray, J. T. (1976). Alcohol and backward masking of visual information. *Journal of Studies on Alcohol, 37,* 40–45.

Moskowitz, H. A., & Roth, S. (1971). Effect of alcohol on response latency in object naming. *Quarterly Journal of Studies on Alcohol, 32,* 969–975.

Moskowitz, H. A., & Sharma, S. (1974). Effects of alcohol on peripheral vision as a function of attention. *Human Factors, 16,* 174–180.

Moss, H. B., Kirisci, L., Gordon, H. W., & Tarter, R. E. (1994). A neuropsychologic profile of adolescent alcoholics. *Alcoholism: Clinical and Experimental Research, 18,* 159–163.

National Health and Medical Research Council. (2001). *Australian alcohol guidelines: Health risks and health benefits.* Canberra: Commonwealth of Australia.

Newcomer, J. W., Farber, N. B., Jevtovic-Todorovic, V., Selke, G., Melson, A. K., Hershey, T., et al. (1999). Ketamine-induced NMDA receptor hypofunction as a model of memory impairment and psychosis. *Neuropsychopharmacology, 20,* 106–118.

Nieschalk, M., Ortmann, C., West, A., Schmal, F., Stoll, W., & Fechner, G. (1999). Effects of alcohol on body-sway patterns in human subjects. *International Journal of Legal Medicine, 112,* 253–260.

Office of the Attorney General. (1994). *Criminal justice (public order) act, 1994, Section 4(1).* Retrieved December 20, 2009, from http://www.irishstatutebook.ie/1994/en/act/pub/0002/sec0004.html

O'Mahony, T. F. (2004). A comparison of alcohol abusers who have and have not experienced blackouts. *European Addiction Research, 10,* 95–98.

Palva, E. S., Linnoila, M., Routledge, P., & Seppälä, T. (1982). Actions and interactions of diazepam and alcohol on psychomotor skills in young and middle-aged subjects. *Acta Pharmacologica et Toxicologica (Copenh),* **50**, 363–369.

Perham, N., Moore, S. C., Shepherd, J., & Cusens, B. (2007). Identifying drunkenness in the night-time economy. *Addiction, 102,* 377–380.

Perry, P. J., Argo, T. R., Barnett, M. J., Liesveld, J. L., Liskow, B., Hernan, J. M., et al. (2006). The association of alcohol-induced blackouts and grayouts to blood alcohol concentrations. *Forensic Sciences, 51,* 896–899.

Pihl, R. O., Paylan, S. S., Gentes-Hawn, A., & Hoaken, P. N. S. (2003). Alcohol affects executive cognitive functioning differentially on the ascending versus descending limb of the blood alcohol concentration curve. *Alcoholism: Clinical and Experimental Research, 27,* 773–779.

Pittler, M. H., Verster, J. C., & Ernst, E. (2005). Interventions for preventing or treating alcohol hangover: Systematic review of randomised controlled trials. *British Medical Journal, 331,* 1515–1518.

Price, D. L., & Flax, R. A. (1982). Alcohol, task difficulty, and incentives in a drill press operation. *Human Factors, 24,* 573–579.

Ryback, R. S. (1970). Aeromedical consultation service case report: Two forms of alcohol amnesia. *Clinical Aviation and Aerospace Medicine, 41,* 930–931.

Sarkola, T., & Eriksson, C. J. P. (2003). Testosterone increases in men after a low dose of alcohol. *Alcoholism: Clinical and Experimental Research, 27,* 682–685.

Schneider, E. W., & Carpenter, J. A. (1969). The influence of ethanol on auditory signal detection. *Quarterly Journal of Studies on Alcohol, 30,* 357–370.

Schuckit, M. A., Gold, E., & Risch, C. (1987). Plasma cortisol levels following ethanol in sons of alcoholics and controls. *Archives of General Psychiatry, 44,* 942–945.

Schuckit, M. A., & Smith, T. L. (2000). The relationships of a family history of alcohol dependence, a low level of response to alcohol and six domains of life functioning to the development of alcohol use disorders. *Journal of Studies on Alcohol, 61,* 827–835.

Schuckit, M. A., Smith, T. L., Anderson, K. G., & Brown, S. A. (2004). Testing the level of response to alcohol: Social information processing model of alcoholism risk—A 20-year prospective study. *Alcoholism: Clinical and Experimental Research, 28,* 1881–1889.

Schuckit, M. A., Smith, T. L., & Kalmijn, J. (2004). The search for genes contributing to the low level of response to alcohol: Patterns of findings across studies. *Alcoholism: Clinical and Experimental Research, 28,* 1449–1458.

Schuckit, M. A., Tsuang, J. W., Anthenelli, R., Tipp, J. E., & Nurnberger, J. I. (1996). Alcohol challenges in young men from alcoholic pedigrees and control families: A report from the COGA project. *Journal of Studies on Alcohol, 57,* 368–377.

Schuckit, M. A., Wilhelmsen, K., Smith, T. L., Feiler, H. S., Lind, P., Lange, L. A., et al. (2005). Autosomal linkage analysis for the level of response to alcohol. *Alcoholism: Clinical and Experimental Research, 29,* 1976–1982.

Schweinsburg, B. C., Alhassoon, O. M., Taylor, M. J., Gonzalez, R., Videen, J. S., Brown, G. G., et al. (2003). Effects of alcoholism and gender on brain metabolism. *American Journal of Psychiatry, 160,* 1180–1183.

Schweizer, T. A., Jolicoeur, P., Vogel-Sprott, M., & Dixon, M. J. (2004). Fast, but error-prone, responses during acute alcohol intoxication: Effects of stimulus-response mapping complexity. *Alcoholism: Clinical and Experimental Research, 28,* 643–649.

Schweizer, T. A., Vogel-Sprott, M., Danckert, J., Roy, E. A., Skakum, A., & Broderick, C. E. (2005). Neuropsychological profile of acute alcohol intoxication during ascending and descending blood alcohol concentrations. *Neuropsychopharmacology, 31,* 1301–1309.

Sierksma, A., Sarkola, T., Eriksson, C. J., van der Gaag, M. S., Grobbee, D. E., & Hendriks, H. F. (2004). Effect of moderate alcohol consumption on plasma dehydroepiandrosterone sulfate, testosterone, and estradiol levels in middle-aged men and postmenopausal women: A diet-controlled intervention study. *Alcoholism: Clinical and Experimental Research, 28,* 780–785.

Simester, A. P., & Brookbanks, W. J. (2002). *Principles of criminal law.* Wellington, New Zealand: Thomson Brookers.

Spear, L. P. (2000). Adolescent period: Biological basis of vulnerability to develop alcoholism and other ethanol-mediated behaviors. In A. Noronha, M. Eckardt, & K. Warren (Eds.), *Review of NIAAA's neuroscience and behavioral research portfolio: NIAAA research monograph No. 34* (pp. 315–333). Bethesda, MD: National Institute on Alcohol Abuse and Alcoholism.

Sprandel, U., Tröger, H.-D., Liebhardt, E. W., & Zöllner, N. (1980). Acceleration of ethanol elimination with fructose in man. *Annals of Nutrition and Metabolism, 24,* 324–330.

Tabakoff, B., Hoffman, P. L., Valverius, P., Nhamburo, P. T., & Saito, T. (1988). Selectivity of ethanol's action on brain receptor systems: Catecholamines and ethanol. *Australian Drug and Alcohol Review, 7,* 39–42.

Tagawa, M., Kano, M., Okamura, N., Itoh, M., Sakurai, E., Watanabe, T., et al. (2000). Relationship between effects of alcohol on psychomotor performances and blood alcohol concentrations. *Japanese Journal of Pharmacology, 83,* 253–260.

Tasmania Law Reform Institute. (2005, March). *Intoxication and criminal responsibility* (Issues Paper No. 7). Hobart, Australia: Author.

Texas tourism officials worried about public intoxication crackdown. (2006, March 31). *USA Today* [Online]. Retrieved December 20, 2009, from http://www.usatoday.com/travel/news/2006-03-31-texas-drinking_x.htm

Tygstrup, N., Winkler, K., & Lundquist, F. (1965). The mechanism of the fructose effect on the ethanol metabolism of the human liver. *Journal of Clinical Investigation, 44,* 817–830.

United Nations General Assembly. (1966, December 16). *International covenant on civil and political rights* (United Nations Treaty Series, Vol. 999). Retrieved December 20, 2009, from http://www.unhcr.org/refworld/docid/3ae6b3aa0.html

Veldman, R. G., & Meinders, A. E. (1996). On the mechanism of alcohol-induced pseudo-Cushing's syndrome. *Endocrine Reviews, 17,* 262–268.

Votava, B. T. (2001). Missouri dram shop liability: Last call for third party liability? *University of Missouri–Kansas City Law Review, 69,* 605.

Wallgren, H., & Barry, H. (1970). *III. Actions of alcohol: Vol. I. Biochemical, physiological and psychological aspects.* Amsterdam: Elsevier.

Walter, R. M., & Noth, R. H. (1984). Effects of alcohol on the endocrine system. *Medical Clinics of North America, 68,* 133–146.

White, A. M. (2003). What happened? Alcohol memory blackouts, and the brain. *Alcohol Research & Health, 27,* 186–196.

Wilhelmsen, K. C., Schuckit, M., Smith, T. L., Lee, J. V., Segall, S. K., Feiler, H. S., et al. (2003). The search for genes related to a low-level response to alcohol determined by alcohol challenges. *Alcoholism: Clinical and Experimental Research, 27,* 1041–1047.

Williamson, A. M., & Feyer, A.-M. (2000). Moderate sleep deprivation produces impairments in cognitive and motor performance equivalent to legally prescribed levels of alcohol intoxication. *Occupational Environmental Medicine, 57,* 649–655.

Wolkowitz, O. M., Reus, V. I., Weingartner, H., Thompson, K., Breier, A., Doran, A., et al. (1990). Cognitive effects of corticosteroids. *American Journal of Psychiatry, 147,* 1297–1303.

World Health Organization. (1992). *The ICD-10 classification of mental and behavioural disorders: Clinical descriptions and diagnostic guidelines* (10th revision). Geneva, Switzerland: Author.

3

The Origins of Drunkenness

Anne Fox

The archaeological evidence suggests that human beings have been intentionally fermenting fruits and grains for at least 12,000 years. However, because alcohol is a naturally occurring substance, it is highly probable that humans were drinking it well before that. But why and how would they have done so? How might our early ancestors have explained and understood drunkenness? How might the chemical effects of alcohol have influenced social interaction? What possible use could drinking have served for early hunter-gatherers? What spiritual and social meanings may have been attached to alcohol? What relevance does this all have to understanding contemporary drinking behavior? Building on Chapter 2 on the biology of intoxication, this chapter introduces an anthropological explanation of the phenomenon of drunkenness and concludes with two illustrative case studies on the tradition of "the round" and drinking among indigenous Australians.

THE EVOLUTIONARY APPROACH: WHAT'S IN THE WIRING?

Although most ethnographers and sociologists acknowledge that nearly every society on earth uses at least one variety of a psychoactive substance (K. Fox, 1999) and that most societies use alcohol, very few studies have ventured beyond cultural anthropology (i.e., situating the reasons and functions for ritualized behavior in the social, national, ethnic, or cultural setting) to delve into the possible evolutionary reasons for these acts. Until recently, few scientists in the current climate of political correctness and creationism were prepared to make forays into the forbidden zones of functionalism and human nature.

Functionalism, the explanation of human behavior based on the utility of its consequences, has fallen out of favor in the social sciences for two main reasons: first, because the logic was flawed—the consequences of an action cannot also be the cause of the action—and second, because much of human behavior, including drunkenness, can be decidedly dysfunctional (for a good treatment of this argument, see Barkow, Cosmides, & Tooby, 1992). There remains also the persistent belief that the human being is born a *tabula rasa,* a content-free mind ready to be programmed and imprinted with the dominant culture in which it is raised. The idea that human beings have an inherent "nature," or hard-wired ways of thinking and behaving, makes many people uncomfortable, as it puts us on the same spiritual level as "soulless" animals. In this persistent paradigm, most human behaviors (e.g., drinking to drunkenness) are seen as purely socially or culturally constructed. However, to say that we behave the way we do because our culture influences us is to make culture the *über* reference to explain all irrational or inexplicable group behaviors.*

The evolutionary view, by contrast, avoids these contradictions and tautologies. The adaptations of human behavior were formed for the Pleistocene world of our hunter-gatherer ancestors, not for the modern context, and many are as out of place now as a horse and cart on a highway. The main premise of this chapter is that drunkenness is explicable in evolutionary terms as a maladaptive behavior that is "functional" only in the sense that it helps us cope with this impossible situation. We should therefore begin our investigation by returning to the Pleistocene.

Why is it necessary to investigate the life of the ancestors of our species—or even, for that matter, the lives of prehistoric peoples? In a nutshell, because *they* are still *us.* The innovations of the past few thousand years may have been life-changing for our species (and our planet), but they have not altered our basic biological makeup, which has been about a million years in the making. Our minds are still adapted to the perils, the stresses, and the joys of life as a Pleistocene hunter-gatherer. If the evolution of the human being were expressed as a 24-hour day, the modern era would barely take up the last few seconds—not enough time to change human nature.

* Anthropologist Adam Kuper (1999) urged us to "avoid the hyper-referential word [Culture] altogether, and to talk more precisely of knowledge, or belief, or art, or technology, or tradition, or even of ideology … appeals to culture can offer only a partial explanation of why people think and behave as they do, and of what causes them to alter their ways" (pp. x–xi).

Think of the dog: Whether it is a Chihuahua dressed in pink and riding in a handbag or a beagle sniffing for drugs at the airport, it is still, at heart, a wolf, a hunting pack animal. The best dog trainers recognize this and exploit the animal's pack mentality to direct its behavior. That, unlike the dog, we are conscious of our own condition (we put on our own collars) does not change the fact that we are as bound as the dog by our evolutionary past. We are primates that just learned a few tricks—and learned to pass those tricks on to the next generation, which then added more tricks. But the tricks (e.g., writing, symbolic thought, central heating, the Space Shuttle program, mobile phones, genetically modified crops, and the electric potato peeler) do not change who we are. They are like the Gucci diamante collar on the Chihuahua: The dog is still a wolf; we are still just a very clever ape.

Drunkenness is a great trick. It allows us to cope with the fact that we have traveled very far from home, far from the environment to which we are naturally suited (called the *environment of evolutionary adaptedness* by modern anthropologists), in which we spent several million years as hunter-gatherers. Drunkenness occurs as a consequence of living *outside* this hunter-gatherer context: Evidence for this, as explored later, is found in the predominance of drunkenness in the modern indigenous hunter-gatherer peoples who have been displaced, corralled, or "disarmed."

However, our natural fit in the environment may have been disrupted some time further back in human evolution.* Evolution is not a linear progression to greater degrees of perfection—it is an imperfect system of trade-offs. In the fading light of the Paleolithic era, the advantages that we had gained over our primate cousins (e.g., language, imagination, and the safety of large groups) came at a high price. For example, we gave up easy childbirth and independent offspring for the advantages of larger brains and bipedalism. When we started to speak, we began to give up direct physical contact as our primary comfort. Imagination (symbolic thought) opens up avenues of invention, but it also delivers terror, ambition, self-delusion, and disappointment. Larger groups are safer, but they are fraught with the anxieties of social complexity: hierarchies, rivalries, jealousies, and aggression. Many of our oddest behaviors can be seen as counterbalancing efforts, attempts to bring us back to a more comfortable,

* I am tempted to agree with Adams (1979/2004), who wrote in *The Hitchhiker's Guide to the Galaxy* that we all had made a big mistake coming down from the trees in the first place.

primeval state. Any action, however odd, that can take us to this state will trigger the reward center of our brains. Drinking alcohol is one of the things we do to make ourselves feel better, feel happier. A brief overview of the chemical and evolutionary origins of what we think of as "happiness" can help us to understand such odd behaviors as drunkenness.

THE PURPOSE OF HAPPINESS

The chemistry of happiness involves a complex set of neurotransmitters that enable us to feel elated, relaxed, euphoric, and even bonded to each other. The best known of these neurotransmitters are the *endorphins* (the word is a contraction of *endogenous* and *morphine,* meaning *internal morphine*). The reward system of our brains that regulates these "free drugs" (e.g., serotonin and dopamine) is triggered mainly by actions that are directly related to our survival. In a nutshell, what makes us happy, or what triggers the internal reward, is what is good for our survival—or, more precisely, what *was* good for our survival in the Paleolithic era.

The things that make us happy are not all about comfort, security, food, and sex: To have survived the brutal world of the African savannahs, early hominids had to be bold, industrious, courageous, competitive, inventive, cooperative, intelligent, and opportunistic.* As our numbers increased and our diet improved, our cognitive capacities grew. However, the advent of language, our increasing intelligence, and our capacity for symbolic thought all produced fresh problems. Drunkenness (or, for that matter, drug use) is part of our unique propensity for illusion and self-delusion (something that all other animals lack), which we employ to deal with our changed world. As anthropologist Robin Fox (2000) put it:

> We are born, digest, reproduce, grow old, and die like animals. And that of course is all there is to it. But the animals get on with it. … We invent incredible fantasy structures to justify our getting on with it (in one way rather than another) and call these *cultures.* … We are the masters of

* These categorizations are adapted largely from anthropologist Desmond Morris's (2004) wonderful book *The Nature of Happiness.* Morris also included several additional types of "negative happiness" such as deriving pleasure from pain (which stimulates endorphins), cruelty (a form of hypercompetitive happiness—literally "beating" rivals), and self-delusion.

illusions. Magicians fascinate us; our hero is the con man. We invent the great con man in the sky to mastermind the greatest illusion of all: That we need not die. And aiding and abetting all this is the prime agent of rationality, the brain, whose major function is to protect us from reality so that we might act and not drown in endless processes of unresolvable decision-making. (p. 46)

ALCOHOL THE TRICKSTER

The ethanol molecule is itself a con man. Simply put, it hits the reward center of the brain, causing a flood of endorphins, thus fooling us into thinking that something good has happened. Alcohol is like an applause button in the brain: Whatever we are doing, add alcohol, and it will feel right. This may go some way toward explain the "400 rabbits" phenomenon—the myriad of behavioral effects that alcohol seems to cause. In fact, it does not *cause* any behavior in particular, but merely rewards whatever the drinker happens to be doing, indiscriminately applauding whatever record is playing.

As seen in Chapter 2, alcohol does have a physiological effect, but the manifestation of this effect is always culturally influenced. Inebriation, like any other state (e.g., relaxation, joy, grief, disgust, or anger), is shaped by the way we are taught to express it. Equally, however, the presence of alcohol in the brain triggers a raft of complex neurological processes, none of which produces carbon-copy reactions in all individuals. Alcohol's perceived effects are so deeply imbedded in our cultural consciousness that they kick in even if we are made to think that we have consumed alcohol. One study found that a mere suggestion that one has consumed alcohol can affect one's memory of events, without any alcohol entering the brain (Assefi & Garry, 2003); and numerous studies have demonstrated that sober individuals who drank an alcohol placebo but believed that they were drinking alcohol behaved, for example, more aggressively or promiscuously than was the norm for them otherwise (Fakjær, 1992; George & Norris, 1991; Giancola, 2002a, 2002b; Giancola et al., 2002; Southwick, Steele, Marlatt, & Lindell, 1981). But we are getting ahead of ourselves. Let us return to the Pleistocene and ask: Were our hominid ancestors aware of alcohol?

HOMO EBRIUS: A TASTE FOR ALCOHOL

Two human features suggest a possible evolutionary basis for our penchant for alcohol: the hereditability of alcoholism and the hereditary variance of levels of the alcohol-metabolizing enzyme *alcohol dehydrogenase* (ADH). Dudley (2000) suggested that the evolutionary origin of human alcoholism lies in our frugivorous (fruit-eating) primate ancestors:

> Olfactory localisation of ripe fruits via volatised alcohols, the use of alcohol as an appetitive stimulant, and the consumption of fruits with substantial alcohol content, potentially characterise frugivorous primates, including hominoids and the lineage leading to modern humans. Patterns of alcohol use by humans in contemporary environments may thus reflect a maladaptive co-option of ancestral nutritional strategies. (p. 3; see also Dudley, 2002)

In other words, a keen sensitivity for the smell and taste of alcohol served our ancestors well, as it helped them to locate ripe fruit, a rich and necessary source of calories and nutrition. In much the same way, the reward center in our brains is triggered when we eat anything with a high sugar and fat content. In an environment where such things were rare, this built-in craving was adaptive: It motivated us to seek them out and consume as much as possible before the supply disappeared. In modern times, however, this craving has become a maladaptive burden.

Alcohol differs from other substances that can be abused in that it is produced by plants as a natural process of fermentation of sugars by yeast, and not as a part of the plant's defense mechanism. Almost all drugs (e.g., cocaine, cannabis, opium, hallucinogenic mushrooms, and caffeine) are derived from plant toxins that are inherently designed to produce strong and adverse reactions. Because alcohol occurs naturally in the body, we have evolved with enzymes to metabolize it. The presence of the ADH enzyme in humans also indicates a long evolutionary history of frugivory.* Without ADH, most ingested food would make us drunk, because some

* Man's very distant cousin, the treeshrew, has been observed to sip the fermented nectar of pollen flowers—a concoction with an alcohol concentration of 3.8% of alcohol by volume. Luckily for the shrew, its alcohol metabolism is far more efficient than that of humans, and this constant bingeing does not result in intoxication (Wiens et al., 2008). Robert Dudley, of the University of California at Berkeley, called this "a beautiful example of the natural biology of alcohol consumption" (quoted in Hecht, 2008, para. 8).

level of fermentation occurs in the intestines. Dudley (2000) explained this as follows: "If regular exposure to low concentrations of ethanol is an inevitable consequence of ripe fruit consumption, then selection will favour the evolution of metabolic adaptations that maximise physiological benefits and minimise any costs associated with ethanol use" (p. 386).

Levels of ADH vary in human populations: Those whose evolutionary past did not include exposure to fruit or grains (e.g., the Eskimo/Inuit and those descended from them, such as the Native Americans and the Japanese) have a genetically lowered resistance to alcohol (lower levels of ADH) in a relatively significant percentage of the population. This suggests that among populations with high levels of ADH, alcohol consumption (either directly or via naturally fermented substances) has existed long enough to effect a genetic change. If we assume that humans originally had quite low levels of ADH,* as there would have been no need to metabolize more alcohol than the body could produce naturally, then for natural selection to have changed our genetic makeup to high-ADH-producing beings would have taken around 400 generations, or approximately 12,000 years (Ehrlich, 2000; Wilson, 1975/2000). We can safely assume, therefore, that deliberate fermentation of alcohol has been around for at least that long.

WHEN WAS THE FIRST HAPPY HOUR?

As alcohol is a naturally occurring substance, and as many animals have been observed to deliberately seek out and eat fermented fruits (with some comic aftereffects), it is highly probable that our early hominid ancestors would also have had some awareness of the side effects of well-fermented fruit. If they did choose to gorge on these themselves, the effects would no doubt have been mild, as, unaided, fruit will only ferment to around 1 to 2% alcohol by volume (ABV). One would have to eat an awful lot of

* Another clue that alcohol consumption was not prevalent in the Pleistocene is the fact that it does not feature predominantly in the list of substances that elicit sickness symptoms in pregnant women. Studies have shown that pregnancy sickness deters women from ingesting foods that contain high levels of toxins that could harm the fetus. But the substances that elicit the nausea response are only those that would have existed in a Pleistocene diet. "Modern" toxins, such as certain drugs, nicotine, and other chemicals, fail to elicit the pregnancy-sickness response, as does alcohol. This implies that alcohol is too recent a substance to have exerted selection pressure for aversion (Profet, 1992).

bad fruit to achieve anything like the state of intoxication that we would recognize today—a badly upset stomach would no doubt have been the result of such an attempt. Would this have put our ancestors off, though? Some hunter-gatherer tribes that still exist today withstand tremendous physical pain (e.g., vomiting and cramps) to achieve an altered state from psychotropic plants.

A number of anthropologists dispute the idea that drinking alcohol could have occurred in prehistoric Europe. Sherratt (1991) argued that the wild fruits available in Europe's primeval temperate climate (including *vitis sylvestris,* the wild grape) would simply not have contained enough sugar to ferment (see also Rudgely, 1994, p. 32). The sugar-rich varieties we use today are the result of centuries of careful selection and forced breeding. Rudgely (1994) and Sherratt (1991) doubted that alcohol was deliberately made before around 3500 BCE.

There are, however, other sources of sugar besides flesh-rich fruit. Honey is one; tree sap is another, particularly sap from the date palm in South Africa (Hornsey, 2003), which has one of the highest concentrated sources of sugar of any plant (up to 70%), and from maple and birch trees, used by the North American Indians. Honey and sap are both still used by contemporary tribes around the world to make alcoholic brews. Archaeological evidence also indicates that sap was stored for future use, so it is likely that some fermented, either accidentally or deliberately (Hornsey, 2003, p. 7). Siegel (1989, p. 117) described prehistoric cave paintings depicting the collection and storage of honey, which ferments easily. South American Indians still use a variety of wild jungle fruits; modern Central Americans use varieties of cacti (as did the ancient Aztecs). The list is endless. And, as mentioned earlier, if animals as large as elephants can become visibly intoxicated from fermented wild fruits on the African plains, why should we not suppose that early man could have done so as well? The arguments to the contrary seem to be motivated by a puritanical reluctance to accept that intoxication is an ancient and very human practice.

Edwards (2000) also fixed on the date of 3500 BCE for the earliest use of alcohol, arguing that even the simple process of gathering fruit, adding water, and waiting a few days for fermentation to begin implies a settled, agricultural way of life. Did our early ancestors have the means to keep old fruit long enough to reap the benefits? The first stone tools date to around 2.5 million years ago. Because many tools have been found alongside animal bones with distinctive cut marks, we can safely assume that systematic butchering of carcasses occurred around this time. It is therefore certainly possible that other skills such as skinning and preparing and using hides, empty gourds, horns, or even skulls as carrying vessels was also existent at this time. If we can accept that *Homo habilis* made receptacles in which to carry fruit and water, then it is not too great a leap of faith to assume that, in a hot climate, the contents of such a vessel could easily have transmuted into a fizzing, fermented concoction.

The earliest members of our lineage (see Figure 3.1), the *australopithecines* (dating from 4.5 to around 2 million years ago), could walk upright, but there is no evidence to suggest that they used fire or stone tools. Evidence from fossil sites suggests that they were more hunted than hunters, falling prey to hyenas, leopards, sabretooth tigers, and other predators (Stringer & Andrews, 2005). Lacking fire, weapons, claws, or large canine teeth, it is unlikely that they would knowingly have incapacitated themselves with fermented fruit juice.

The first members of our own genus, *Homo* (including also *Homo habilis, Homo rudolfensis,* and *Homo ergaster*), appeared between 3 and 2.5 million years ago and were better protected by tools, weapons, and fire—they may have been the first drinkers. A strategic switch from primarily gathering food to cooperative hunting heralded a new era of success for our ancestors. However, hunting in the Pleistocene environment could be highly dangerous. It required intense cooperation, concentration, communication, planning, and strategy, all capabilities that were really only possible in ever larger and larger groups. When food sources were located, these also had to be defended, often from other aggressive primates. Very early in our evolution, it became hard-wired into our brains that the group was the source of survival. Being separated or ostracized from the group meant death. So, from very early on in our prehistory, drinking, if it occurred at all, would be strongly associated with the group. The act of preparing and sharing a fermented beverage does indeed imply a greater complexity of social organization than was probably found among *Homo habilis,* but late *Homo erectus* and early *Homo sapiens* definitely had the capabilities—large group size and control of fire, both of which could have enabled group members to spend "leisure" time in relative safety. But the question again is this: Why would they drink?

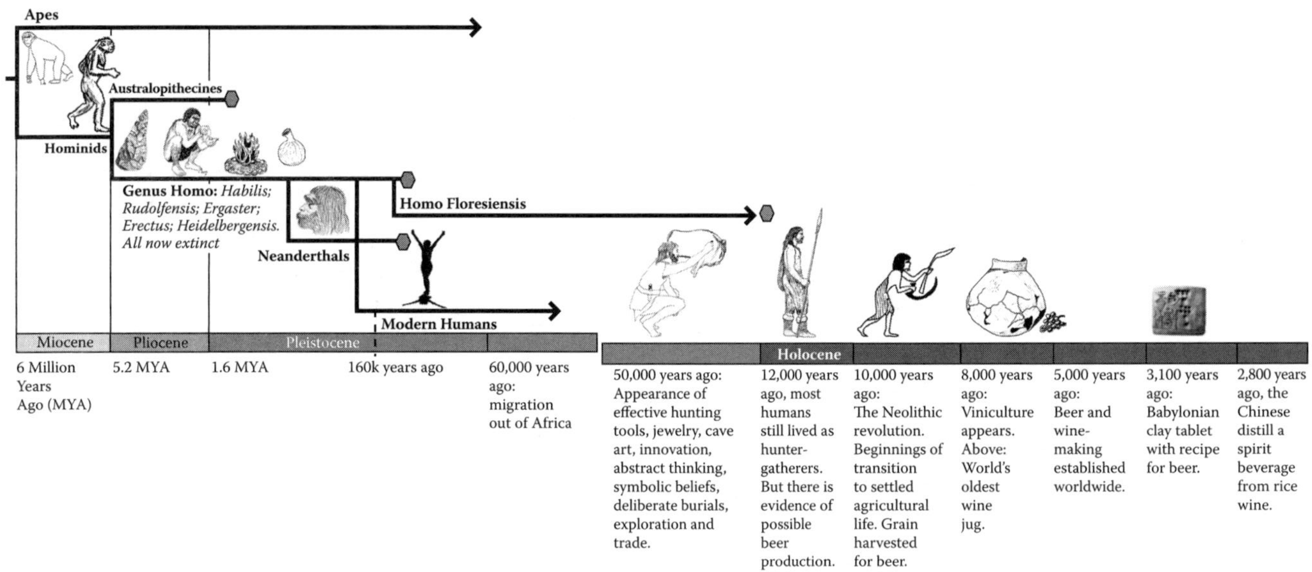

FIGURE 3.1
Human evolution and alcohol.

ALCOHOL AND THE LANGUAGE BARRIER

If we look at the effects of alcohol on the brain and the benefits that this might provide to humans, it is hard to imagine any good reason for our very early forefathers to imbibe. The raw material for the *Homo* species is a primate adapted to living only in small groups, with a brain capable of dealing with the complexity of only a handful of relationships. For larger groups, however, among *Homo erectus* and early *Homo sapiens,* alcohol's unique properties may have been advantageous. The universality of alcohol as a symbol of trust may provide a clue as to its possible original use. The expansion of human groups was necessary for survival, but it came at a price.

The main method of bonding used by all our primate cousins is grooming. When chimpanzees groom each other, their brains are flooded with endorphins, the feel-good chemicals. When we hug and touch each other, we experience similar feelings. If relationships, comfort, and touch were not rewarding, we might not have survived to create the large groups that we needed for our existence. It is hard-wired into us that we need other people, we need to be part of a group, and the chemical system in our brains reinforces this with every touch. The feeling of belonging to and being accepted by a group is one of the most powerful of all human desires, driving much of what we do.

The problem with grooming, though, is that it is very time-consuming: Studies of chimpanzees have shown that they spend almost 25% of their time at it. (To relieve group tensions, bonobos take grooming to extremes and engage in casual sex up to a dozen times a day.) As anthropologist Robin Dunbar (1997) theorized, when human groups "outgrew" grooming—that is, when group size exceeded around 40 individuals—something else was needed to maintain social cohesion. Again, we capitalized on something we probably already had: vocalizing. When chimpanzee groups are separated, as when they forage large areas or nest at night, they "chorus," calling out to each other constantly. A beneficial accidental modification in the primate larynx enabled some of our ancestors to refine the primate vocalizing into coherent sounds that could express more than gestures, grunts, or hoots. We could now bond ever larger and larger groups through talk. Human language, Dunbar argued, is grooming at a distance. Even now, with all we have to talk about, around 70% of all human conversation is social.

Again, however, the solution was not perfect. There is a problem with language. This innovation, which was probably responsible for our success as a species today, has a major flaw: It cannot do the one thing that grooming does, which is to cause a physiological response, a pleasurable, physical, rewarding feeling that causes the release of that flood of endorphins. And it still can only really be done properly in small groups. According to Barrett, Dunbar, and Lycett (2001), "Language is such a poor medium for expressing our inner feelings that most of us resort to good old-fashioned primate mutual mauling when it comes to building more intimate relationships" (p. 328).

One of our solutions was to make language *feel* more like grooming. We have several ways of doing this. One is through laughter. Laughter creates a *physical* response to speech: When we laugh, our brains flood with endorphins and a group of chemicals called *catecholamines,* which make us feel relaxed and help us trust the person who is speaking. Consequently, we spend an awful lot of our time (and money) trying to make each other laugh. Another way is to modify the voice itself to elicit more of an emotional response, through singing or oration. And yet another way is through drink.

Building on Dunbar's argument that language is grooming, it is my theory that alcohol has evolved, in almost every society on earth, as a social substance important to group bonding (or group synchronization) because it makes verbal communication feel more like grooming, and so increases trust. When drinking in a group, we often actually touch our glasses, a symbolic connection that takes the place of touching each other. Before the invention of mugs or glasses, it could be speculated that the use of animal horns as vessels would also lead to sharing drinks: You cannot put a full horn down but you can pass it around. The endorphins that are released in the brain when one drinks can be seen as a mirror, an imitation of the feelings one gets when one is groomed, hugged, kissed—when one is getting those wonderful rewards of belonging and of intimate connection with another human being. Alcohol can therefore actually make language physical by simulating grooming. It is really no wonder that it is a substance that has probably been used throughout our late evolutionary period by our ancestors and into the Holocene, the modern age.

IN VINO VERITAS: ALCOHOL AND TRUST

There is another problem with language: It opens up opportunities for deception. Whereas it is quite difficult to truly "fake" affection or submission with physical gestures, it is easy to deceive with language, demonstrated by the fact that we tend to use expansive hand gestures when we are trying to convince someone of the veracity of our words or feelings. Again, what we see here is an evolutionary trade-off. Large groups are great for safety but dependent on cooperation. Cooperation needs rules and policing: The larger the group, the more opportunity for freeloading and cheating. The cost and benefits of language and group sharing have led to what some have termed an evolutionary cognitive "arms race," culminating in our finely honed mental ability to detect cheats (e.g., Brown & Moore, 2000; Cosmides & Tooby, 1992; Trivers, 1971). Our fascination with magicians, con men, and tricksters stems from our preoccupation with detecting the deceivers in our group. We devote inordinate amounts of time (and gossip!) to freeloader detection. If trust is of prime importance in a tightly bonded group, it is even more important when members of such a group encounter strangers. Interaction between strangers, even 20,000 years ago, is evident from the fossil record, as stones, skulls, amber, and other objects are often found hundreds of kilometers from their origin.

Finding out if someone is trustworthy or a cheat can be a lengthy process, but what if there was a shortcut to trust? Alcohol has properties that can help us overcome the flaws in language design. Warburton (1999) found that alcohol slightly alters the way in which our brains "hear" and process words, particularly words that have threatening overtones (e.g., *cancer*): It lessens the brain's reaction to such words, thereby making conversation a far less anxious task. Drunkenness also reduces the ability to be deceptive and to detect deception (Bradley & Ainsworth, 1984). Added to the simulated grooming effect of the endorphins, these features help to facilitate the feelings of bonding and trust between drinkers.

Contemporary research into attitudes toward drunkenness shows that many modern drinkers believe that alcohol reveals a "true" self, free of cultural constraints (McDonald, 1994; Winslow & Hall, 2006). In some cultural settings, the drunk is believed to be the voice of truth (sometimes painful) for an entire community. For example, Dennis (1979), in describing the role of the drunk in Mexican villages, concluded that

> apparent inebriation serves to define a crucial role in village life: the licensed drunk pierces the elaborate information-control devices of the community and provides the barefaced facts and opinions which normally go unspoken. Like the fool in a Shakespearean play, the Oaxacan drunk is accorded the special privilege of speaking the truth. (p. 64)

Alcohol works not only with words but with emotions, too. Magnetic resonance imaging (MRI) brain scans reveal that, when sober individuals are shown photographs of frightened faces, the amygdala lights up the screen, indicating an emotional response. In people whose blood alcohol concentration is over 0.8 mg/ml (the legal limit for driving in many countries), however, this part of the brain is less responsive, showing equal reactions to frightened and neutral faces. In other words, alcohol could be said to suppress our natural anxiety around other individuals (Gilman, Ramchandani, Davis, Bjork, & Hommer, 2008). Some have reasoned that, as one's ability to perceive threats diminishes, he or she is more likely to become aggressive. However, as reduced ability to identify threatening behavior in another person is coupled with the pleasurable feelings associated with alcohol's activation of the brain's reward center, this could equally explain why the majority of people are less aggressive, rather than more, after drinking. Studies have also shown that others really do appear more attractive to those who are drunk (Parker, Penton-Voak, Attwood, & Munafo, 2008). Clearly, these effects of alcohol could have been useful in interactions between people.

A SUPERIOR WEAKNESS: ALCOHOL, STATUS, AND STRENGTH

Trust is important to the group, but so is the display of strength and superiority. Paradoxically, among males of many cultures, drinking to drunkenness is taken as a sign of strength and manliness. According to Zahavi and Zahavi (1997), intentionally and obviously handicapping oneself may be a way of signaling to rivals and predators that one is actually more powerful than appearances would suggest. If the signal is outrageous enough, the predator is likely to think it is genuine and not waste any energy on the chase. Think of the peacock's tail: Such an obvious encumbrance should have spelled swift death for peacocks in the wild, yet they survive. Diamond (1991/2004), in his book *The Third Chimpanzee*, gave another example: a gazelle that, instead of fleeing as fast as it can, leaps straight up and down into the air when approached by a stalking lion. In addition to possibly discouraging predators, such ostensibly self-destructive signals also serve as indicators of fitness to females of the same species: Bright plumage, long tails, and extremely risky behavior all signal to them that the male has survived despite his handicap and must therefore be genuinely strong.

Extrapolating from Zahavi and Zahavi's (1997) *handicap principle*, Diamond (1991/2004) speculated that chemical abuse and other risk-taking by humans can be partly explained by the same principle: Incapacitating oneself with alcohol (or drugs) sends a signal of superiority to both rivals and potential mates. Group incapacitation through drink also serves as a warning to freeloaders that the benefits of group membership come at a price. As Butler (2006) noted in her research among the Quichua speakers in Ecuador, drinking to intoxication with one's peers sends a strong signal that one is willing to sacrifice one's person and surplus resources (e.g., time or money) to maintain group cohesiveness: "The belief that alcohol ritually shared created unbreakable social ties sanctioned by God and other spirits served as a warning against the likelihood of new *compadres* receiving the benefits and refusing the enduring obligations of the exchange relationship to which they had publicly committed" (p. 235).

All of these features—increased trust, the physical sensation akin to grooming, and the use of alcohol as a signal of strength and group loyalty—may explain why alcohol became more and more attractive to early human groups.

HUNTER-GATHERER CULTURES AND DRUNKENNESS

Intentional drunkenness implies several things: planning, foresight, and creation of vessels to prepare the beverage in the first place; strong group cooperation to achieve this; groups large enough to guarantee the safety of the drinkers, or a safe dwelling or structure in which to drink; and stratification, either social or based on age or gender, as it is unlikely that all members of a pre-Neolithic group would become drunk at the same time. Having demonstrated that it would be possible, I think, it is unlikely that drinking to drunkenness would have occurred before the advent of what anthropologists call *behavioral modernity.*

If we could find alcohol consumption among the existing hunter-gatherer groups today, we could presume that the practice has more ancient origins; if we cannot, then it is more likely that alcohol production and consumption is a phenomenon of the Neolithic revolution. As such, I argue that it is most likely a result of the rise of religion and of the increasing need for methods of group cohesion. Surveying the existing hunter-gatherer tribes of the world, little evidence is found of deliberate fermentation of fruits, grains, or vegetables. Apparently, most hunter-gatherers today procure alcohol from neighboring agriculturalists (Tanaka, 1980). Among these hunter-gatherer tribes, however, we find a strong propensity for achieving altered states through psychoactive substances (see discussion in Case Study 3.2 on the use of *pituri* by Australian Aborigines). We can assume that these practices have a more ancient origin. An altered state would have required an explanation, and that explanation undoubtedly led to the realm of belief—belief in forces unseen. Once we begin to see such beliefs emerge (e.g., as evidenced by deliberate burials around 75,000 years ago), we are on the verge of behavioral modernity, the point at which *Homo sapiens* began to demonstrate symbolically based behavior. Behavioral modernity also encompasses many features of "humanness" that persist to this day: Large groups, permanent dwellings, social hierarchy, and belief in other realms are features of what we know as *culture.*

Cultural diversity abounds in nearly every category of comparison among the existing hunter-gatherer and forager groups (e.g., the Australian Aborigines, the Inuit of the Arctic, the Ache of Paraguay, the Ati of the Philippines, the Hadza of Africa, and the Shoshone of the Great Basin, to name but a few). Presumably, tribes of prehistoric times were even more diverse in their ways, but, despite this variety, hunter-gatherer and forager groups display some key similarities: lack of personal possessions, a high value placed on reciprocity (and food sharing), egalitarianism, and male–female divisions of labor (Panter-Brick, Layton, & Rowley-Conwy, 2001). In many hunter-gatherer societies, one also finds beliefs concerning the sacredness or magical properties of certain liquids—water (as it is life-sustaining), liquids emanating from the body (blood, sweat, milk, semen), and substances created from the juice of plants. With the high value placed on reciprocity and food sharing, it is most likely that, if our ancestors used fermented beverages, the drinking cultures would have been molded within these parameters—sharing of special liquids. Early differences could also have been found in the beliefs surrounding alcohol's powers. Were these powers believed to be supernatural? Were the fruits from which the alcohol was produced viewed as the very flesh of the Gods, as was believed about certain hallucinogenic plants? Was the effect of alcohol seen as the result of spirit possession? Or was alcohol merely regarded as a mundane terrestrial food source? These differences may have been instrumental in shaping the drinking cultures of the societies that formed from these early groups.

All in all, a picture may be emerging of sparse use of alcohol by our early ancestors for social bonding, to indicate trust between group members and strangers, and possibly for displays of male prowess. The Neolithic revolution, however, would significantly transform the way we drank, leading to the development of drinking cultures, our next subject.

THE EVOLUTION OF DRINKING CULTURES

The Rise of Culture

Before we proceed with our investigation into the evolution of alcohol consumption and drunkenness as part of human cultures, we need to clarify the meaning of the term *culture*. Many authors have reduced its definition to merely the social transmission of information (e.g., Boyd & Richerson, 2005; Mace, Holden, & Shennan, 2005). Then other primates also have cultures, however—even groups of chimpanzees have their own ways of cracking nuts or fishing for termites that are distinct from neighboring troops. Only in human culture is symbolic information passed on. We alone are conscious in the sense of being able to remove ourselves from our context and consider why things are and how they might be otherwise. Not only can we fantasize, but we have the intelligence and skills to reconstruct our reality based on our fantasy. We alone among primates can imagine and pretend: We can imagine we are somewhere else or pretend we are someone, or even something, else.

We are a species adapted primarily for a subtropical climate. Without culture, we could not have populated all areas of the earth. As such, culture is part of our survival mechanism. A lone individual, in a foreign land with a different climate and ecology to her own, would not survive long if she had no one to teach her the local ways: how to steer clear of poisons and predators; how to find food, water, and shelter; how to keep warm or cool; and so on. Much cultural information is thus critical to our survival—so critical, in fact, that we encode much of it in religious belief systems that ensure compliance through fear of punishment by deities. Other aspects of culture are not so obviously useful. Although such things as marriage customs (e.g., monogamy versus polygamy) may seem to be matters of choice, when placed under scientific scrutiny, they are also explicable in terms of the best reproductive fit to the environment and its resources (Barkow et al., 1992).

Cultural differences act as markers of group identity: "On the basis of relatively few pieces of key information on language, dialect, and customs, you could probably identify the origins of most human beings to within a few hundred miles" (Mace et al., 2005). As we are a territorial species that forms relatively small and tightly bonded groups, it is in our nature to differentiate ourselves as much as possible from rival groups. Deliberate cultural differentiation may also be a driver of cultural variety. Despite its dazzling variety—and its darkest horrors—human culture is the expression of human nature.

Some anthropologists have likened culture to a living coral reef that grows on a submerged structure: Each reef has its own living characteristics, but it is still shaped by the structure beneath it. So beneath the dazzling festival of different cultural practices is a very human structure, and this can be seen in cultural features that are common to all human societies. All humans are, after all, the same species, and although we do things in different ways, there are some constants. As Barrett et al. (2001) put it, "The rules that guide human behavior are relatively simple and—more importantly—are universal. The complexity of human behavior derives not from these rules but from the wide variety of demographic, ecological and social environments in which individual humans seek to apply these rules" (p. 381). Some of the rules and features that almost all human cultures have in common, as R. Fox (1991) wrote, are:

> rules about property; rules about incest and marriage; customs of taboo and avoidance; methods of settling disputes with minimum bloodshed; beliefs about the supernatural and practices relating to it; systems of social status; initiation ceremonies; courtship practices involving adornment of females; symbolic body ornaments; generally speaking, activities set aside

> for men from which women are excluded; some form of gambling; tools and weapon making industries; myths and legends; dancing; various doses of adultery and homicide; suicide; homosexuality; schizophrenia; psychosis and neurosis, and various practitioners who take advantage of or cure these depending on how they are viewed. (p. 276)

It is, in fact, part of our nature to make rules about everything! To the preceding list, however, I would add the use of intoxicating substances. Siegel (2005), in *Intoxication: The Universal Drive for Mind-Altering Substances,* even argued that, following the human drive for food, sleep, and sex, intoxication is the "fourth drive." But is it really just a drive for intoxication? Is there not some other explanation beyond the simplistic notion that humans just like to get wasted?

Group Bonding and Drunkenness

Regardless of their size, organization, political system, or religion, human groups need to overcome social anxieties through bonding. Although group-bonding methods differ across cultures, there are many features that recur consistently and can be considered universals of human bonding. The most obvious of all these is what anthropologist Chris Knight (1990) called the *ritual synchronization of emotions,* devising ways of getting large groups of people to do the same thing at the same time, especially accompanied by rhythmic movements (e.g., dancing, singing, chanting, or drumming). Performing activities that involve rhythmic movements done in synchronization with others causes a release of endorphins. Repetitive motion, especially when practiced as a group, has thus become a powerful feature of all human societies. There is not one tribe, not one society on the face of the earth, that does not have some form of ritual synchronizing of group emotions, be it drumming, dancing, chanting, twirling, marching, praying, singing, clubbing, or raving. For our hunter-gatherer ancestors, the ability of many people to move as one body would have provided a distinct survival advantage: To animals, groups of humans in synchronized movement appear as one frighteningly large animal. Safety in numbers is thus enhanced.

The ritual dances in which almost all indigenous hunter-gatherer peoples engage serve two key functions: to practice synchronized hunting moves and to encourage cooperative behavior in the group. Through a series of experiments, Wiltermuth and Heath (2009) confirmed what tribal elders and military instructors have known for centuries—that behavioral synchronization, such as simply walking in step with others for a brief period of time, results in more cooperative and unselfish behavior.* This effect of enhancing the cooperative urge occurred equally strongly whether the behavioral synchronicity involved motor activities such as marching, rowing, and dancing or more social activities such as singing. Wiltermuth and Heath concluded that "synchrony rituals may have therefore endowed some cultural groups with an advantage in societal evolution leading some groups to survive where others have failed" (p. 5).

In post-Neolithic "modern" societies, many of these group rituals were suppressed or relegated to a few times a year. In the absence of such activities, however, humans are still driven to synchronize—thus, group drinking may have served as a substitute. Chemically speaking, alcohol may better enable us to synchronize our actions due to another peculiar effect called *alcohol myopia.* Repeated experiments have found that individuals under the influence of alcohol, when faced with multiple choices or cues in their surroundings, develop an intense focus on what they believe to be the most important thing (Fillmore & Vogel-Sprott, 2000; Steele & Josephs, 1990). This also appears to enhance the ability to perform repetitive, rhythmic motions. Group drinking not only facilitates synchronization of activity but is also a synchronized activity in itself. Turmo (2001), in describing male drinking in the taverns of Andalucía, Spain, observed that, "Amid the conversation, each person concentrated on his glass, drinking more quickly or sipping more slowly, as everyone tried to sustain a more or less homogeneous rhythm in the number of orders" (p. 136; see Case Study 3.1 at the end of this chapter for a description of *the round,* a synchronized drinking ritual found in many societies).

Obviously, geography and ecology influence a group's physical cohesion: Seas, mountains, rivers, forests, and deserts all contribute to unique microclimates to which particular groups become adapted for survival. Many other elements play a part in keeping things together, however. Table 3.1 depicts several of these cultural elements and the role that drinking or drunkenness may play in enhancing them.

* Recent advances in neuroscience have also confirmed that the urge to copy or synchronize our behaviors seems to be built into the brain in the form of mirror neurons that are activated when the individual either performs an action himself or sees someone else performing it.

TABLE 3.1

Alcohol Consumption and Group Cohesion

Group Cohesion Method	"Benefit" of Alcohol Consumption/Drunkenness
Kinship and marriage: Built-in strategies for belonging	Even in prehistory, alcohol might have served as part of a "bride price." The effects of alcohol are also pertinent to courtship, attractiveness, and sex. Drinking is, and has long been, a central feature of weddings.
Social rules: Enforced by those of high status and also by social contract (e.g., marriage)	By being a symbol of trust, a shared drink can seal a verbal contract.
Cultural remission	Most societies on earth include several forms of *cultural remission*—that is, relaxing the rules of normal behavior. Alcohol provides the medium that makes much of this possible. Drunkenness also provides individual drinkers with an excuse to break the social rules without retribution.
Group synchronization rituals: The ritual synchronization of emotions, such as through dancing, singing, or performance of sacred rites	With drunkenness comes the effect of alcohol myopia, which enhances the drinkers' focus on repetitive action and enables a feeling of merging, unity, and oneness.
Initiation rites	Alcohol and enforced drunkenness are used in many rites of group initiation around the world.
Physical touch and displays of affection	Drunkenness, in many cultures, allows for the physical expression of affection that would normally be proscribed, especially between men.
Exchange/reciprocity	As a symbol of trust, wealth, and happiness in many cultures worldwide, alcohol serves as the ultimate gift. Gift exchange (reciprocity and indebtedness) is a major force in social cohesion.
Sharing/cooperation	Humans are an altruistic, cooperative, sharing species. This evolved as part of our survival strategy. Drinking in groups can formalize and enable acts of sharing and cooperation.
Gossip/social conversation	Language evolved primarily as a tool for social cohesion. Alcohol is a feature of many social gatherings: It has a pronounced effect on the way the brain processes words, lowering anxiety.
External threat	A real or perceived external threat can bind a group together. Alcohol is a feature of many warrior cultures.

(continued)

TABLE 3.1 (CONTINUED)

Alcohol Consumption and Group Cohesion

Group Cohesion Method	"Benefit" of Alcohol Consumption/Drunkenness
Beliefs: Shared beliefs, particularly regarding the origins of the group, have a powerful influence on group cohesion	Alcohol is an integral part of many belief systems; drunkenness, in some belief systems, is a manifestation of spirit possession.

Alcohol and the Neolithic Revolution

Whatever the patterns of drinking were among our earliest hunter-gathering ancestors, there is little doubt that they would have changed during the period that historians call the *Neolithic revolution.* Archaeological finds show that, by the upper Paleolithic (around 40,000 years ago), human life had made a dramatic shift away from the nomadic, egalitarian, small-scale world of the hunter-gatherer. More and more evidence emerges of permanent dwellings, domestication of animals, small-scale farming, net fishing, and other industrious activity. Items such as jewelry found in burials begin to indicate a degree of social stratification: Some individuals were becoming more important than others. What difference did these changes make, and how might they have influenced the consumption of alcohol?

Contrary to popular belief, the farming life is far more labor intensive than hunting and, in terms of yield per person, far less rewarding. Nor is it any healthier: Studies of the bones of the first farmers and coexisting hunter-gatherers show greater prevalence of disease among those choosing the settled life (Cohen & Armelagos, 1984). So why was there a rapid worldwide shift to this life of servitude?

One widely accepted explanation is a period of global warming and drought that depleted the predictable supply of wild foods. Once the sedentary farming lifestyle had been established, it required a commitment, a form of enslavement to the soil, that could not be easily reversed. Others have pointed out, however that, despite these climatic changes, many people managed to remain hunter-gatherers, so some other force must have been at work. Mithen (1996) wrote that, "While sedentary farming may represent a poorer quality of life for a community as a whole, when compared with a mobile hunting-gathering lifestyle, it provides particular individuals with opportunities to secure social control and power" (p. 255).

With farming came a new phenomenon: surplus food. A surplus in a community creates problems: the need for a guardian for the food, storage facilities, and, inevitably, a concept of property and ownership. With ownership, come power structures, rules, and regulations, all of which are hard to undo. The convergence of these changes suggests that scarcity of resources caused by climatic change resulted in greater competition for resources and for control over them.

As Morris (2004) put it,

> the delicate balance between competitiveness and cooperation was disturbed, swinging in favour of increased competition. The larger populations in the ancient towns and cities had become more impersonal. Bonds of friendship were being loosened. Those individuals who became local leaders were able to use their power with more ruthlessness than before. Slave classes emerged. For the majority, happiness went into sharp decline. (p. 18)

Although the agri/herding life possibly provided greater safety and stability, it was boring when compared with the hunting-gathering lifestyle. Millions of years of evolution had primed our brains for excitement, change, risk, and challenge. Hunting could result in daily thrills and nightly celebrations and reenactments of triumph. Unlike the hunter-gatherers, who sat down to share meals on most nights, the agriculturalists could only do so within the time frames allowed by those in power, or the tyranny of the planting and harvesting timetable. Thus, it is possible that the first "binge" culture was born. It is arguable that the modern worker who goes out every night (eating, dancing, drinking, and socializing) is unconsciously trying to re-create the happier Paleolithic conditions that we are born to expect. A study of the Mambila people in Nigeria and Cameroon (Rehfisch, 1987/2003) offers an example of how settled agricultural life leads to demarcations of work and play: "The day-to-day routine is highly repetitive and acknowledged by the Mambila to be boring. It is only during the festive seasons that excitement reigns and life is lived to the full" (p. 143). So it is possible that the settled, agricultural life both precipitated the need for stress relief and supplied the means.

Neolithic Alcohol Production

Although our early ancestors may have used fruits or sap to make alcohol, the advent of grain cultivation brought with it a new source of alcohol. There has been an ongoing debate among anthropologists about the motivation for the cultivation of grains in the first place: Was it to produce bread or beer? (Braidwood et al., 1953; Katz & Voigt, 1987) The staple food of almost all humans is now some form of grain, derived from primitive grasses. Although we take this for granted, Ronald Good, an eminent British botanist, begged a question: "Growing plants whose fruits are large and conspicuous is understandable—but grasses?" (quoted in Hornsey, 2003, p. 9). Hornsey (2003) spelled out in great detail how the two most commonly domesticated cereals, wheat and barley, are nutritionally deficient in their raw form to other food sources available at the time: They are low in protein, fats, minerals, and B-group vitamins. To make matters worse, they contain phytates, phosphorus compounds that inhibit the absorption of other key elements in the body. Yet many of these deficiencies are reversed or improved by malting, allowing the grain to germinate before fermenting so as to release the necessary enzymes. This process also dramatically improves the taste of the cereal and its stability for storage purposes.

Harlan (1967) found that the mature seeds of wild grains such as those grown in the Near East could easily have been harvested, ground with stones, mashed, boiled, and fermented, employing similar methods to those used by contemporary African tribes with domesticated grain, to produce a weak but nutritious and flavorful beer. Evidence of all the materials necessary for this process (e.g., sickle blades, stone pounding and grinding tools, and storage pits) has been found at Natufian sites in the southern Levant and ancient sites in Syria and Turkey dating from 12,000 years ago. Although, as noted earlier, some historians doubt that brewing could have occurred before the invention of pottery, as boiling water in other organic containers (e.g., wood or skins) is too difficult (for review, see Hornsey, 2003), if alcohol production did occur this far back in our history, it is likely that it contributed to the development of cultures in which drunkenness was a ceremonial and regular occurrence. If the methods used were anything like those found in contemporary African tribes (as is likely), the production of the substance must have been inherently ritualistic. For example, among the Bantu people of South Africa, the production of sorghum beer is a 5-day process that results in a brew of around 2 to 4% ABV, which has to be consumed within 2 days. The marriage of ritual and drinking is still entrenched in many African societies; as one Tanzanian put it, "If there's no beer, it's not a ritual" (Willis, 2002, p. 61).

"Civilized" Drinking

The evidence of organized beer-making in ancient Egypt dates back to the Predynastic Era (7500–5100 BCE) and possibly even earlier in the Near East, in the Sumer region of Mesopotamia (Hornsey, 2003). Although ancient civilizations differed greatly in terms of the beliefs and attitudes toward alcohol, the theme of a divine, transformative substance permeates the mythologies. The ancient Egyptians regarded drunkenness as a near-sacred state, which is not surprising considering that, in Egyptian mythology, mankind would have perished at the hands of the wrathful goddess Hathor had it not been for the calming effect of beer (Hathor's hangover, however, brought the first sickness to the world).

The Aztecs also believed alcohol to have a divine origin: Mayahuel, the goddess of the maguey plant (which yields the alcoholic drink *pulque*), and her husband Patecatl, the god of healing and fermentation, gave birth to 400 (meaning "innumerable" in ancient Aztec) divine children or "rabbit gods," collectively known as Centzon Totochtin, the gods of drunkenness, each a patron of a different manifestation of drunkenness. Today, some older-generation Mexicans still spill a few drops of *pulque* to the master of them all, Ometochtli, or Two-Rabbit, the god of fertility and wind, and say of a drunkard's unusual behavior that "he has become his rabbit," both testimonies to the endurance of mythological beliefs (de Rojas, 1998; Mitchell, 2004). Mitchell (2004) suggested that the "tradition of expecting the unexpected set the stage for a rapid acceptance of the Spanish notion that drunkenness mitigated responsibility for even the gravest sins" (p. 13), an attitude that is still widespread in Mexico.

For the ancient Greeks and Romans, wine was a crucial element of both social and religious rituals. Dionysus, the god of wine (and, later, the Roman god Bacchus), was the conduit for human ecstatic madness and communication with the dead. He was also called Eleutherios, or the Liberator, for his ability to free a person from his or her ordinary self, again, a belief about alcohol that persists in many drinking cultures today. According to Hajar (2000), the etymology of the word *alcohol* most probably derives from the Arabic word *al-kol* or *al-ghol* (from which we derive our English word *ghoul*), which translates simultaneously as either a shape-changing genie (or spirit) or a substance that can take away or cloud the mind.

One of the earliest written records illustrating beliefs about alcohol in ancient civilizations comes from one of the oldest literary epics in the world, *The Epic of Gilgamesh,* written nearly 5,000 years ago. The story, in a way, mirrors the journey of the "wild" hunter-gatherer toward the "civilized" life. Interestingly, alcohol features prominently in the process. In a nutshell, the story goes like this: Gilgamesh was a terrible king, a tyrannical ruler, and thus he offended the gods, so they decided to challenge him by creating a man who was as strong and powerful as he was. Out of mud and clay, they created a primitive, bestial, apelike creature called Enkidu. Enkidu was completely "unsocialized" in the ways of humans: He grazed on grass and milked animals and could not even speak. Gilgamesh discovered the existence of this creature and decided to tame him. He did this by sending out Shamat, a prostitute,* to find Enkidu. Shamat slept with Enkidu for 7 nights, so he became calmer, and then she began to instruct him in the ways of humans:

> The harlot spoke to Enkidu saying: / "Eat the food, Enkidu, it is the way one lives. / Drink the beer, as is the custom of the land." / Enkidu ate the food until he was sated, / he drank the beer—seven jugs!—and became expansive and sang with joy! / He was elated and his face glowed. / He splashed his shaggy body with water, / and rubbed himself with oil, and turned into a human. (Kovacs, 1989, p. 16)

So, in a reversal of what is commonly believed today, in at least one ancient civilization, alcohol turned the beast into a man. (It should be noted that, with an intake of seven cups of beer at one sitting, Enkidu would qualify by current standards as the first binge drinker in recorded history.) Similarly, in Homer's *The Odyssey,* drinking alcohol was a mark of civilization, a proof that man had risen above the bestial state exemplified by the lawless one-eyed Cyclops, who, like Enkidu, lived wild in caves.

* Although most translations label Shamat as a prostitute, anthropologist Robin Fox (*in press*) pointed out that she "is actually a priestess of the goddess Ishtar. These priestesses, representing the goddess, had intercourse with men who gave gifts to the temple, much as happened in ancient Judaic ritual, and still happens in parts of southern India, where the practice is known as *devadasi.*"

The sentiment that we have been "raised" up out of brutish animal nature by civilization, expressed in *The Epic of Gilgamesh* and *The Odyssey*, is still popular today. As "civilized" life took us ever further away from our pre-Neolithic state, beliefs began to emerge that it was civilization itself that created modern man in all his power and glory. This notion has been at the foundation of our sciences for centuries, as Rousseau (1762/1968) wrote in *The Social Contract* in 1762:

> And although in civil society man surrenders some of the advantages that belong to the state of nature, he gains in return far greater ones; his faculties are so exercised and developed, his mind is so enlarged, his sentiments so ennobled, and his whole spirit so elevated that ... he should constantly bless the happy hour that lifted him for ever from the state of nature and from a narrow, stupid animal made a creature of intelligence and a man. (p. 64–65)

The most common belief about alcohol found in many cultures today, however, and one of the reasons why the substance is feared and regulated, is that alcohol can reverse this process: It can strip back the protective barriers of civilization to reveal violent, stupid, brutish nature underneath. In contrast, the anthropological viewpoint is that what alcohol reveals is not our savage or primitive nature, but our very cultural and "civilized" essence. Farming, social stratification, and political and state governing structures have all contributed to the development of drinking cultures that are based on ritual and power. However, alcohol is not an inert substance like money or cloth. It has the power to create or facilitate a dramatically altered state—for this reason, its use has long had religious or magical connotations.

Alcohol and Religion

In many cultures, alcohol is not only a passage to the realm of the dead, but a link to the spiritual world through an offering of drink. De Garine and de Garine (2001) described a legend of the Tupuri people in Northern Cameroon in which death itself began with drunkenness, when drunken villagers were mistaken for the dead and buried. Ancestor worship is prominent in the Dupa religion of Northern Cameroon. The spirits of the dead are given offerings of *bumma* (fermented sorghum or millet beer) throughout the year. Death does not release a person from craving beer: The cause of illness among villagers is often diagnosed as an ancestor's craving for *bumma* (de Garine & de Garine, 2001, p. 197).

Many societies have institutionalized alcohol to the point where communication with the spiritual world is impossible without it (two other liquids, water and blood, often share this ability to bridge the physical and the spiritual; Akyeampong, 1996). A number of the hunter-gatherer cultures surviving today still integrate psychoactive substances into their beliefs, using them to induce a dream state and reveal knowledge of the spiritual world. Early man had no scientific way of interpreting dreams, and these fanciful creations that occur as a by-product of neural information processing may have seemed very real to our ancestors. If these dreamlike visions could also be produced by ingesting a substance, it might have been assumed by early humans that something of the hidden realm—some power, force, or spirit—was contained in the drink.

As we have already established, deliberate drunkenness would only be safe in groups that are large enough to protect those who were incapacitated. These large groups would probably have given drinking a special time-and-place significance, and rules surrounding alcohol use would most likely have developed. For example, if it was believed that a spirit or spirits entered a person through the drink, it would make sense to forbid it to pregnant women for fear that such possession might harm the unborn child. Lewis-Williams and Pearce (2005) argued that in the Neolithic revolution, social stratification, with its inherent inequalities, was as much a result of the rules of early religion as of population pressures and other factors. The propensity to have vivid dreams, visions, and hallucinations is not universal—some people are more likely than others to have "visions" or to experience altered states of consciousness. The greater the ability, the more these people would consider themselves (and would be considered by others) to be closer to the realms of the unseen and therefore distinguished from ordinary people. Lewis-Williams and Pearce provided evidence to suggest that, in the Neolithic, "new values entered human ethics," and "access to 'spiritual' states was regulated" (p. 58). With access to sacred sites regulated, temples and magical places became open only to those who had the authority of a connection with the spirit world—and any substance that provided a bridge to this world would also begin to be regulated.

Although its use may have been controlled, many of the world's belief systems and religions have traditionally celebrated alcohol as a gift from the gods. Early Christianity was no exception, although many of the original songs of praise to alcohol have been adulterated in translation. For example, in the Gutenberg Bible, a familiar line in Psalm 23, in Latin, reads as:

> … *et calix meus*
> inebrians
> Quam praedamus est!

This literally translates as "and how beautiful is the cup that makes me drunk!" The King James translation, however, altered this passage to "my cup runneth over," thereby glossing over all reference to drunkenness and the pleasures of wine as a gift from God.* Today, drunkenness is taboo in many religions, punishable by stoning, flogging, imprisonment, or other sanction. What differentiates cultures that celebrate drunkenness as a connection to the gods from those that view it as an abomination against them? How can we explain this from an evolutionary perspective?

I suspect that the prohibitions on alcohol by many of today's religions have their origins in the control of female sexuality, rather than concern for spiritual purity. A universal problem for all male primates (including humans) is how to ensure paternity of offspring. A mother knows her children; a father can never be sure. Because it is part of our genetic hard-wiring to invest the most energy and resources into our own offspring and closest relatives, it is an in-built male imperative to control the reproductive process as closely as possible. Among the great apes, the solution is the control of females by dominance of one male who earns mating rights to an entire harem. Modern humans have adopted a variety of mating strategies, the most common worldwide being polygamy (one husband, several wives). The most common to Westerners is serial monogamy through pair-bonding (having only one wife or husband at a time). Polyandry (one wife, several husbands) does occur but is very rare. Interestingly, where it does occur, the husbands rarely live with the wife or look after her children, preferring the greater genetic certainty of looking after their sister's children. It would seem at first glance that pair-bonding

* I am indebted to anthropologist Robin Fox (personal communication May 19, 2009) for providing this insight.

is the most egalitarian of all systems. A cursory glance at adultery laws the world over, however, would prove otherwise:

> Until recently, essentially all such laws—Hebraic, Egyptian, Roman, Aztec, Moslem, African, Chinese, Japanese, and others—were asymmetrical. They existed to secure a married man's confidence in his paternity of his children, and for no other purpose. … No criminal law against male infidelity even existed until a French law of 1810, and that law only forbade a married man to keep a concubine in his conjugal house against his wife's wishes. (Diamond, 1991/2004, p. 80)

Even in the most modern democracies, the drive to control female sexuality is still present. It is not difficult to understand, therefore, how alcohol came to be viewed as a threat in many societies: Alcohol enhances the sexual response in females by increasing testosterone; it reduces anxiety and makes faces more attractive (Parker et al., 2008); culturally, it is often associated with uninhibited behavior—clearly, this is not a substance that is safe to have around in paternalistic societies that are dominated by the fear of female infidelity. Although humans may have a drive to bond, celebrate, and experience transformation, the evolutionary game is, after all, about reproduction. The alcohol laws, prohibitions, and taboos that are present in many of the world's holy books may have developed in response to the need for control—control of female sexuality and, after the Neolithic revolution, control of the lives of peasants, serfs, and workers (see also Chapter 4).

Cultural Remission

There is a constant tension in all primate groups, including our own, between the need to ease social anxiety and the need to sustain the tension that creates the anxiety in the first place. We are a hierarchical and competitive species. Even in the smallest, most intimate groups, we compete for mates, status, resources, territory, and power. Any substance that can "magically" dissolve this structure will undoubtedly be viewed as both desirable and dangerous. Its use must be carefully regulated lest things fall apart. And yet we are driven, at least periodically, to dissolve the structure and feel unified and homogenous, as one people. We have numerous ways of doing this, as previously described, but, when other outlets become unavailable, group drinking serves as a perfect substitute.

Many of the drinking cultures that persist to this day could be viewed as simultaneous examples of conformity to the status quo (because we are, by nature, conformists) and rebellion against it (because the status quo is incompatible with our Palaeolithic mind). Many of these forms of "rebellion" are also sanctioned by the dominant powers. As Mitchell (2004) wrote:

> Civilizations are not built on coercion alone; the dominant know they must return at least a small portion of the energies they capture. In any number of ancient urban cultures, the monopolization and timely redistribution of alcohol supplies figured as importantly as religion itself in establishing new power relationships and hierarchical mindsets. (p. 14)

So, ironically, the forms of rebellion (or *cultural remission*) through drink are often interpreted by anthropologists as merely reinforcing the social order.

Drunkenness can be seen as an example of Turner's concept of an *antistructure* activity, which, as Abrahams explained in his foreword to Turner's (1969/1995) *The Ritual Process,* applies to "all confrontative activities, especially those drawing on a refashioning of self through masking, costuming, acting in a predictably disorderly fashion" (p. x).

As nation states developed, and human groups expanded into ever larger communities, the outlets for group-bonding activities were further and further restricted. Larger groups and societies lost the natural methods of group bonding inherent in small groups; yet, the larger the group, the greater the need for formalized or ritualized expressions of belonging. Communal bonding rituals have both fascinated and terrified rulers and religious institutions for millennia. There is a great threat to hierarchical power inherent in a crowd's ability to feel and act as one. Yet, activities that achieve this ecstasy of communal bonding continue to surface in all cultures. It can be seen, for example, in carnivals, rock concerts, modern sports crowds, raves, nightclubs, and evangelist religious gatherings—Durkheim (1912/2008) called this *communal effervescence,* and Turner (1969/1995) described it as a *ritual of communitas,* a transformational group experience. The intensity, frequency, and temperament of such activities—as well as the character of the drinking cultures that surrounded them—have been shaped over centuries by geography, climate, and sociopolitical shifts among peoples.

Drinking Cultures in Europe

Recent comparative studies divide drinking cultures into two broad types: the *wet* and the *dry drinking cultures.* Wet cultures, also described as *integrated, moderate,* and *nontemperance,* are characterized by the integration of drinking into everyday situations, where drunkenness is not necessarily the goal of activities (Levine, 1992; Raitasalo, Knibbe, & Kraus, 2005). Here, alcohol is generally thought of as a food substance without transformative powers; drinking patterns, however, are under strict social controls that curb overtly drunken behavior. In dry cultures, also referred to as *nonintegrated, immoderate, temperance,* or *ambivalent,* alcohol consumption is normally segregated to specific times and places, and drunkenness often features as the main aim of drinking. The term *ambivalent* refers to the paradoxical coexistence of heavily proscriptive rules and laws regarding drinking on the one hand, and a permissive and tolerant attitude to drunken behaviors on the other (Campbell, 1991; Room & Mäkelä, 2000). In Europe, some authors make a geographical divide between the two styles:

> There has been a long-lasting view of a north-south gradient of drinking and binge drinking, with a higher integration of drinking in everyday life (e.g., drinking with meals) in southern Europe, and stronger traditions of ostensive drunkenness in northern Europe. (Kuntsche, Rehm, & Gmel, 2004, p. 122)

Engs (1995) attributed the development of these two types of drinking cultures to past links with either the Roman or Germanic traditions. The regions that were either gradually absorbed into Roman civilization or forcibly colonized by Romans still maintain the "southern" or wet style of drinking, whereas regions that resisted Roman rule persist with the Nordic, Germanic style of drinking. Climate might have also played a role: It is possible that drinking cultures characterized by heavy drinking and episodic displays of drunkenness are those that developed in northern regions with shorter harvest times and, thus, fewer occasions to access alcohol, whereas the more relaxed attitude persisted in milder, more fertile climates of southern Europe. The features of these two cultures are summarized in Table 3.2.

It must be noted that drinking in many European countries exhibits a mixture of the features described in Table 3.2; moreover, patterns change over time, with heavy drinking often accompanying rapid socioeconomic change.

TABLE 3.2

Roman and Germanic Drinking Cultures

Features	Roman Drinking Culture	Germanic Drinking Culture
Climate and habitat	Hot weather climate, longer agricultural season, largely deforested regions	Cold weather climate, shorter agricultural season, heavily forested regions
Feasting traditions	Regular feasting throughout the year with an abundance of wine (Cunliffe, 1988)	Sporadic feasting, shaped by a scarcity of resources and seasonal availability of alcohol; tradition of "feast drinking" (Cunliffe, 1988; Engs, 1995)
Access to alcohol	Egalitarian access to alcohol among rich and poor	Hierarchical access to alcohol
Predominant type of alcohol	Fermented: wine	Brewed: ale

For example, Purcell (1985) found that the Romans enjoyed a brief period of drunkenness during rapid expansion of urban centers and compared this to the rise of drunkenness in the United Kingdom during the industrial revolution. Recent change in some societies from an integrated or wet culture to dry or ambivalent culture has been blamed on the export of culture through global media and "alcotourism," the bad behavior of tourists from heavy-drinking cultures. These shifts, however, could also be a reflection of internal changes in many southern European societies away from traditional, seasonal agricultural patterns to more urban working rhythms.

MODERN DRUNKENNESS: THE HOLOCENE HAPPY HOUR

Social Stress and Drinking

Laboratory experiments consistently show that drugs and alcohol appeal particularly to stressed animals (e.g., Miczek, Hubbard, & Cantuti-Castelvetri, 1995; Vengeliene et al., 2003). Rats kept in dark, overcrowded conditions or isolated from their kind will consistently choose alcohol and even heroin over food and water (Geller, 1971). Until recently, it was assumed that it was the addictive potential of the drug itself that caused the drive to consume and that, unless restrained, any rat or monkey (and, by inference, any human) would self-administer the intoxicating substance to the detriment of its health. In a series of experiments, however, Alexander (2001) overturned some of these assumptions by re-creating the classic addiction experiments, but with unstressed animals: He built an environment that mimicked perfect rat living conditions (in terms of space, activity, and the ability to build nests and mate). In these experiments, although some rats tried the drug, they consistently rejected it in favor of plain water; even previously addicted rats stopped using when placed in this environment. In other words, animals living in or close to their environment of evolutionary adaptedness do not have an appetite for drugs. This would appear to be a basic mammalian pattern: Humans are no different.

Since the Neolithic, in many societies, there has been a continuous dissolution of small tribal communities, combined with urban crowding and stress. Encountering strangers used to be the exception to daily life—now it is the rule. The larger and more complicated societies become, the more we must deal with strangers rather than kin. Anthropologist Kate Fox (2008) discussed the peculiar human sense of unease around social interaction in her book *Watching the English*. Some cultures, notably in the United Kingdom, suffer more from what she called the *social dis-ease* than others and construct elaborate rituals to overcome the anxiety. Alcohol features prominently in many such cultures. Although drinking practices and beliefs differ widely across the globe, the use of alcohol as a symbol of trust has led to the convergence of many drink-bonding practices. In Case Study 3.1 on the tradition of the round at the end of this chapter, French anthropologist Véronique Nahoum-Grappe described one social ritual used in many cultures to overcome this discomfort in social situations and to strengthen bonds among drinkers.

Much as alcohol can make language feel like grooming, it can make fantasy feel like reality. For example, in most cultures, solitary drinking is seen as problematic or is even a taboo. However, in our modern times, when so many people in the industrialized nations lead isolated lives, solitude is the norm rather than the exception. During an informal investigation into reasons for solitary drinking, I encountered many drinkers who used alcohol to enhance their own fantasies. As one single man in his 40s said, "When you are sober, you know that your pillow is just a pillow; but when you are drunk, you still know it, but it just feels easier to imagine it is a beautiful woman who loves you. It makes it just that little bit more real, for a moment."*

Alcohol is often described as a "transformative" substance by drinkers, helping us make the transition from one state to another, or from work to nonwork. The drinking place itself becomes a kind of alternate reality where one can reconstruct oneself as one wishes, apart from the stressors of everyday life (Mandelbaum, 1965; Rooney, 1991). Douglas (1987) described one of the key functions of ritual—and of drinking—as the construction of an "ideal world" (p. 11), whereas Rudgely (1993) wrote of "the universal need for liberation from the restrictions of mundane existence," which can only be satisfied by experiencing "altered states of consciousness" (p. 7).

Social groups under stress tend to drink more, as do groups in which bonding is necessary for survival (or perceived survival). Such groups include soldiers, immigrant workers, fraternity students, sports teams, and adolescents. Young people who do not have clear social structures within which to experience group bonding (and who have not yet developed the social confidence to bond with others) may use alcohol to overcome social stress. K. Fox (2004) argued that young people in the United Kingdom (as in many Western countries) "are not formally 'welcomed' as fully-fledged members of our society until *after* they have struggled through puberty" (p. 364). Deprived of clear-cut rites of passage, young people are left to invent their own rituals to mark their own self-evident transitions in sexual status. These usually involve, according to K. Fox (2004), "getting into trouble for illegal drinking, experimenting with illicit recreational drugs, shoplifting, graffiti-spraying, joy-riding, etc." (p. 364). In societies where there is no clearly divisible youth culture, and in which adolescents are afforded adult status through clear rites of passage, adolescent substance abuse is far less common.

Drinking Among Displaced Hunter-Gatherers

That drunkenness is a consequence of our lives outside the hunter-gatherer context is evident in the predominance of drunkenness in those hunter-gatherer peoples who have been forcibly displaced, corralled, or "disarmed"—for example, Native Americans, Papua New Guineans,

* Correspondence with anonymous respondent.

Australian Aborigines (see Case Study 3.2 at the end of this chapter), and others. Their move from the hunter-gatherer lifestyle to a settled, horticultural existence was like a speeded-up version of the transformations of the Neolithic. These cases should be of particular importance to anthropologists, as they describe in a microcosm the plight of all humans: We are all displaced hunter-gatherers.

The high rates of drinking among indigenous or aboriginal peoples are a pressing problem in many nations. It appears to be a common phenomenon worldwide that members of former hunter-gatherer tribes, and particularly men, are unusually prone to addiction and excess where alcohol is concerned. The subject of much debate for decades, explanations are numerous. Some, such as a genetic vulnerability to alcoholism among certain indigenous peoples and protest drinking against colonial oppression, are discussed in the case study on indigenous Australians at the end of this chapter. The explanations examined next include the displaced warrior phenomenon, traditional "wild man" behavior, drunkenness as male power failure, and cultural patterns of bingeing or feasting.

Displaced Warriors

Cultural change can occur as a result of natural drift or of externally imposed forces. In both cases, however, certain elements of the culture can be retained like a palimpsest, underlying the new beliefs and practices. For example, ritualized forms of aggression and a *macho ethos*—that is, a belief in the supreme importance of male honor and the defense of that honor (or reputation) to the death, if necessary—are particularly prevalent in warrior cultures. In the recent past of many indigenous tribes, killing another man was, at most, a prerequisite to manhood and, at the least, a mark of honor and status. In modern society, however, with the exception of state-sanctioned war, killing another person for the sake of one's own status is prohibited and labeled as murder. However, although modern societies may try to replace traditional tribal warfare with more symbolic forms of killing (e.g., through sports), the cultural norms of machismo and honor can persist. Young men will always need outlets for aggression, especially within cultures where machismo is ingrained in the values. Where no socially sanctioned outlets exist, raw aggression and violence will likely erupt under the guise of some form of madness, drunkenness being the most common. In his study *Weekend Warriors: Alcohol in a Micronesian Culture,* Marshall (1979) described warlike societies that have been corralled, displaced, and introduced to alcohol. Drunkenness became for them a substitute for communal joy, ritual, and, particularly, aggressive male displays associated with war and courtship.

Drunkenness and Wild Behavior

Warrior societies gave high status to wild behavior, because *berserkers* (Norse warriors), *crazy dogs* (groups among Plains Indians), or *wild pigs* (in New Guinea) could be dangerous and intimidating to the enemy through their reckless violence. Such wild men who could work themselves up into a state of killing fury were highly valued. The introduction of alcohol coincided with the loss of this outlet for these men, and the result was often a substitution of wild drunkenness for the formerly adaptive and directed aggression.

The "wild man" can still be found in modern warrior societies. Modern armies may still value the highly aggressive male if, in peacetime, he can be contained. Pierson (1999) identified soldiers he called "natural killers" whom he defined as:

> a person who has a predisposition to kill—he enjoys combat and feels little or no remorse about killing the enemy. These men have existed throughout the history of warfare, and their feats have often been hailed as heroic. They constitute less than 4% of the force, yet some studies show that they do almost half of the killing. (pp. 60–65)

In my research on drinking among Army soldiers in the United Kingdom, I noted several such hyperaggressive and unpredictable characters in the infantry platoons I was following. Although a constant worry to the chain of command for off-duty wild drunken behavior in the towns, a platoon sergeant summed up the usefulness of one such soldier: "He might be a nightmare in the barracks, but he'll be a leader on the battlefield" (A. Fox, in press).

Drunkenness as Male Power Failure

Drunkenness among males of a warrior group can also occur for the opposite reason to that just stated. The truly powerful high-status aggressive male may drink when he has no outlet for aggression; but equally, the downtrodden, low-ranking male could use drunkenness as an attempt to gain a reputation as an unpredictable and formidable fighter. In my field work, I also noted that soldiers who had failed to achieve any status within the platoon ("power failures") often turned to alcohol and to wild-man antics in an attempt to retrieve at least some kind of a reputation. It rarely achieved the desired effects: They were just labeled as sad drunks.

In hunter-gatherer tribes, the wild-man rituals referred to earlier also allowed low-status, stressed, or frustrated males to engage in a "temporary insanity," which served as a "dramatic performance in which individuals may manipulate the public image of themselves" (Marshall, 1979, pp. 112–113). It may be argued that the high rates of drunkenness among males of certain displaced and colonized hunter-gatherer groups today are a widespread enactment of such rituals. McKnight (2002) and others have noted that it is the males of a hunter-gatherer group who are the most deeply affected by the loss of tribal hierarchies, land rights, hunting, and warfare. The fighting men among the Truk Islanders that Marshall studied, the Australian Aborigines, the American Indians, and others have all been made power failures by the colonial state.

Hunter-Gatherer "Binge" Culture

Although the drunkenness that occurs among hunter-gatherers today can be interpreted as the result of displacement, it could also play on a facet of traditional hunter-gatherer culture: Consuming all that is available is the norm among such tribes; as the environment provides all that is needed, there is rarely any surplus or need for food storage.

Binge eating in the modern day tends to involve high-calorie, high-fat, and high-sugar foods. These are the things that, in our past, were in short supply. When they were found, they were quickly and avidly consumed. The biggest hit to the reward center of the brain happens after we eat such substances, leading to the problems of food addiction and obesity we find in our fat- and sugar-rich modern world. We have a built-in propensity for bingeing on certain substances; perhaps in part because of its high sugar and calorie content, alcohol is one of our binge favorites.

Within the hunter-gatherer groups still in existence today, it is easy to see how many have quickly developed cultures of drunkenness. Within other societies, however, as layers of past history and beliefs are encrusted onto the world's cultures, it is far harder to see clearly how some of the modern world's groups came to adopt drunkenness. Traditions cling to the generations; maladaptive patterns creep in and take hold.

Cultures of Drunkenness

Drunkenness often has a different symbolic significance in a society than drinking. So we could say that there are *drinking cultures* and *drunkenness cultures*. What features or characteristics differentiate the two? One possibility is that the extent of drunkenness as a feature of a drinking culture is to some extent predictable in proportion to the distance the population can be said to have moved from the hunter-gatherer lifestyle, as measured by the following: group cohesiveness, cooperativeness, and egalitarianism; outlets (traditions) for expressions of communal joy or ecstasy and synchronicity (e.g., communal dancing); harmony with the natural environment; an active lifestyle; attachment-style parenting of young children (e.g., long duration of breastfeeding and cosleeping); inclusiveness of young adults in adult society (and clear rites of passage that confer adult status); and ritualized outlets for male aggression and competition. There are, however, fairly universal features of the hunter-gatherer lifestyle that, when transposed into a modern setting, can contribute to heavy drinking. My survey of drunkenness cultures (aligning, in some respects, with the traditional wet versus dry assignations, as outlined earlier) has led me to tentatively suggest a list of features that are associated with such cultural traditions:

- Strict demarcation of work and play and a Calvinistic attitude to work.
- Belief in spirit possession or behavioral transformation through alcohol.
- Stark social and economic inequalities.
- Childrearing practices that instill a sense of fear of strangers and that emphasize independence in early childhood.
- The agricultural features associated with episodes of heavy drinking (e.g., short growing seasons and colder climate).
- Displaced, disarmed, or corralled indigenous population.

- Traditions of excess consumption (in many cases, after colonization, indigenous peoples with such traditions transfer these cultural precepts to drinking).
- A warrior culture (or being descended from a warrior culture).

Semper Ebrius? Cultural Shift and Cultural Change

As noted earlier, however, cultural features that shape drinking and drunkenness do change. Cultures change through several mechanisms: branching, borrowing or blending, and innovation—however, these are holistic changes in society that gradually force an accumulation of alterations in behavior. Piecemeal tinkering with peripheral aspects of alcohol consumption (e.g., licensing hours, alcohol price, and age restrictions) is unlikely to bring about major cultural shifts. The "export" of the British heavy-drinking style to other European countries is often cited as an example of cultural change, but, for a drinking style of one nation to be adopted by another, the practice would still have to fit within the parameters of the new environment. Kate Fox (personal communication December 21, 2009) has argued that some societies seem to have a greater "cultural immunity" than others to such external influences. By contrast, if the undesirable aspects of one society's drinking patterns can affect another culture, might it not be possible to "import" moderate Mediterranean-style drinking into the United Kingdom? Can we engineer shifts in drinking cultures? Many anthropologists would say no. As Gusfield (1996) stated, "Grafting a device or activity from one culture to another is itself assuming a consistency of meaning from one subculture to another" (p. 259).

To achieve change in a drinking culture, one must first gain a thorough understanding of the culture itself, its meaning, and origins. Cultural engineering is to anthropology what chemical engineering is to chemistry. It is the practical application of social, biological, and behavioral theory with the aim of effecting change that is willingly accepted by the group in question. To achieve this, one must understand what cultural patterns and precepts are hard-wired into social behavior. For example, although many culture critics predicted that the mobile phone and the computer would turn us into a society of recluses, alienating us even further from the human community, according to anthropologist Kate Fox, they, in fact, achieved the opposite: Their popularity stems not from the excitement about the new-age technology but from their appeal to our stone-age brains—they allow us to stay in constant touch with members of our tribe. In a world where family and tribal connections have become fragmented and tested by distance, the Internet and the mobile phone give us a virtual campfire. Similarly, a deeper understanding of the evolutionary drivers for drinking, especially group drinking, is likely to result in more realistic and lasting changes than knee-jerk or ad-hoc reforms based on what is seen by policymakers as the proper behavior. Interventions may encourage and reinforce so-called *deviance disavowal,* or provide excuses for bad behavior, and perpetuate the belief that alcohol *causes* it. Changing this belief, as Room (1980) concluded:

> involves undoing one of the most durable legacies of the temperance movement, and it is no light undertaking. By now the power of alcohol to make a person mean, vicious and violent is deeply entrenched in song, story and consciousness. Such a redefinition is thus a matter for a sustained campaign of consciousness-changing, and not for a season of thirty-second television spots. (p. 10)

Young people want transformation: As long as they continue to be told and to believe that there is a power in the drink to transform them, drunkenness will persist.

CONCLUSION

So what does all this tell us? A colleague once accused me of suggesting that the solution to alcohol misuse is for humans to go back to wearing skins and sitting around campfires—the "spear-chucker solution" that would have us return to the hunter-gatherer state. Attractive as this might seem (to anthropologists, at least), it is very obviously neither feasible nor desirable for modern society. However, a better understanding of who we are, where we came from, and what we need can help us design social policy that is aligned with, rather than at odds with, human nature. For example, group drunkenness in the United Kingdom could be seen as a Saturday-night nuisance that reflects a breakdown of the social order—or, from an anthropological viewpoint, it can be interpreted as young people engaging in strictly choreographed self-sacrificial

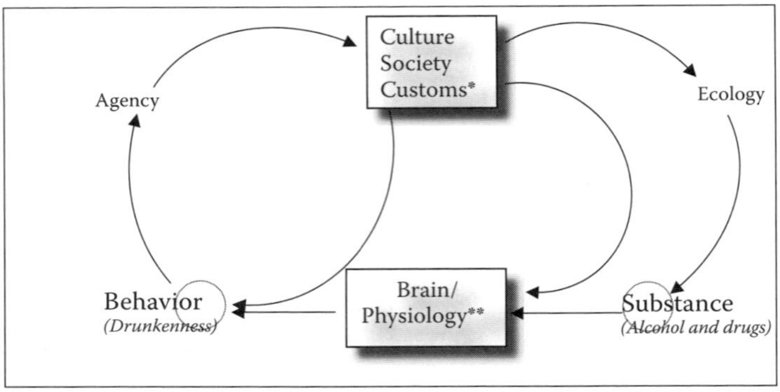

FIGURE 3.2
Interplay of influences on drunkenness. Note: *This includes social norms, values, pre- and proscriptive rules, and procedures. **This includes both so-called hard-wired (e.g., male bonding for hunting/war; aggression for status) and soft-wired (e.g., learned patterns of introversion or gregariousness that can influence the expression of solitary vs. social drinking) dispositions.

group-bonding and mate-attracting rituals within the modern-day hunting grounds of the city center. Among human groups, there will always be a need and drive for communal expressions of joy, solidarity, male competition, rituals of mate selection and sexual signaling, young people's desire for rites of passage and achievement of adult status, and facilitators (whether through custom or substances) for group bonding. When these are absent, uncontrolled, or made unacceptable, alcohol misuse is nearly inevitable.

Alcohol consumption provides a type case for the biosocial study of social action (see Figure 3.2). It involves a natural substance, culturally modified and ingested in customary ways, with well-known physical effects on the brain and physiology of partakers. The partakers' response, however, is determined in culturally prescribed ways by a combination of the brain effects and custom-directed pressures—this produces drunken behavior, which, through individual agency, then reacts back on the social group and affects its cultural values and practices. As this process moves through time, it becomes the *history of alcohol consumption.* As few of the points in this process are static (including, in the past, ecological availability of the substance and, in modern time, the variety of available substances), the whole social tableau moves through time like a ship dragging anchors. Drinking cultures do shift, but not necessarily though the alteration of any one anchor point in this dynamic process. The effects of alcohol on the brain cannot be treated as a kind of "black box" that can explain all behavioral effects and actions. Above a certain instinctive level, human behavior is entirely dependent on the information going through the brain, the learned patterns, the expectations, and the beliefs—all of which shape drunkenness.

Throughout this chapter, we have looked at drunkenness as an important social communicator, used for bonding, relief of stress, and promotion of group solidarity. To understand drunkenness in human society, we must understand, on the one hand, our acquired evolutionary predispositions—universal constants, the human needs, the adapted mental and emotional capacities and predispositions that we have—and, on the other, the particular historical and cultural contexts and circumstances of drinking. We, in fact, know a great deal about both; the insights lie in the interplay between the two. Unfortunately, the anthropological voice gets lost amid monocausal notions about the "inevitable" results of drinking and the relationship between alcohol and behavior. Alcohol encapsulates our most ancient and deep-rooted longings for safety, belonging, praise, transformation, and joy. Drunkenness is an ancient lament.

CASE STUDY 3.1: The Round: Alcohol and Social Connection—An Anthropological Approach

Véronique Nahoum-Grappe

One drinking practice historically rooted in Europe and prevalent in all social classes in many countries is that of *the round,* when drinkers, mostly men, buy each other rounds of alcohol (Nahoum-Grappe, 1991; Nahoum-Grappe, Tsykounas, & Fillaut, 1998). In certain circumstances, one "must" offer a drink, and one "must" not refuse to drink—it is a question of honor and not, perhaps, of pleasure or a compulsion to drink. The round usually takes place at the end of the day or at night, possibly in connection with a meal, in a bar or a restaurant. Despite the more or less festive or cordial context of the round, the predominant mechanism at work is the obligation to reciprocate.

RECIPROCITY

Lévi-Strauss (1967) described a typical scene at a restaurant where the tables are placed very close to one another. How do perfect strangers who are not eating together but find themselves in each other's company coexist? In the exchange of wine, acted out in this scene, the great French anthropologist saw an illustration of the rule of reciprocity, or the obligation to return that which has been offered by another.

> The situation of two strangers facing each other, less than a meter apart, from the two sides of a table in a cheap restaurant is mundane and episodic. However, it is eminently revealing. … It is customary in our society to ignore people whose names, occupations, and social class are unknown. But, in the small restaurant, … people find themselves placed for an hour or so in close proximity and are momentarily united by identical preoccupations. An internal conflict … arises in both parties between the norm of solitude and the fact of the community. … It is to this fleeting but difficult situation that the exchange of wine brings resolution. (pp. 69–70)

Commenting on this and other texts, recent debate among anthropologists takes up the question of the gift and the nature of a collective culture (Descombes, 1996, pp. 162–164; for a review, see Godelier, 1996; Mauss, 1923–1924). The point here is that, under those circumstances and in that particular setting, the exchange just described would not have taken the same direction as an offering of water or tea. Of interest to the ethnologist is the notion of discomfort—the drive of not wanting to lose face is at the heart of public interactions (Goffman, 1974, 1975). Two factors are at work: first, the anxiety of presenting and establishing oneself in society (particularly marked among adolescents); and, second, the social act of reciprocity, obliging the one who has received a gift to give something in return. Defined by anthropologists as being one of the primary conditions for "making society," this free, nonmarket exchange is at the center of numerous theoretical debates.

The first factor—the drive to overcome the social anxiety to present oneself—assumes a consensual value of positivity accorded to alcohol over other substances: Wine offered calls for wine in return; cordiality demands cordiality. An offer of forming a connection, however fleeting, an invitation "to have a drink" allows one to bring resolution to the feeling of discomfort that arises in certain social situations where the ease of being oneself is threatened. The cigarette, the cell phone, and finally the glass of wine, accepted and offered, are some of the socially elegant ways to overcome anxiety. The offering of alcohol is a deliberate and displayed invitation to establish "principled cordiality." It allows and organizes the unspoken recognition of possible discomfort and offers the means for mutual understanding.

The second factor is the collective necessity of the counter-gift, a circular exchange where each person within a group receives and offers something to drink at least once. Why does the modern-day adult feel obligated to reciprocate when given a gift, a sentiment characteristic of nonmarket exchanges? Two trains of thought apply here. First is the functionalist approach, where the role of social drinking is to help adjust the distance between strangers confined to physical proximity within a context where other rituals for interaction fail. The second approach is anthropological, looking at alcohol as the privileged object of exchange, valued above other substances. The custom of rounds offered by groups of drinkers, usually men, occasionally engaged in drinking competitions, illustrates quite well this necessity to give something equivalent (or even better) in return for the first gift.

The description of the scene by Lévi-Strauss presumes that the cordiality implied in the offering of a drink goes without saying. Yet something more is at work: Could the a priori cordiality of the invitation "to have a drink" be linked to the symbolic value of the beverage alone? Wine and other alcohol beverages, gold and jewelry, cakes, sweets, and fine foods are without a doubt the objects often chosen to be offered as gifts to others in our contemporary modes of civility. In France, the bottle of wine is one of the most frequent gifts presented when one is invited to a meal. The value of alcohol as a gift and counter-gift item is in that it deliberately changes the ambiance of the situation and directs it toward cordiality, relieving the discomfort and signaling the offer of social connection. The round can, therefore, be defined as a tactic implemented by the group to manipulate the mood of its surroundings and to imbue it with positivity, even temporarily, for the time of the round.

The psychoactive, inebriating value of any alcohol beverage then comes into play. Perhaps the collective risk-taking of potential intoxication, inherent in the gift and counter-gift of alcohol, is used as a sign of trust or an offer of disarmament. To raise a glass of wine to others, to make a toast, while smiling, seems to be the exact inverse body position to brandishing a weapon. However, the logic of the graceful exchange also obliges you to accept a drink for every gift you offer. It would be an insult to refuse or to express excessive interest, and the cycle of obliged cordiality by the drinking exchange remains fragile.

The bond of reciprocity involving alcohol can be forged anywhere people get together. The offer to "have a drink" is a classic shortcut to better relate to someone to whom one has no connection. If the counter-gift of alcohol allows everyone to save face, it is because this offering is an invitation to nonaggressive connection between strangers: Words, laughter, and civilities can then be exchanged as well, gradually cementing the bond between strangers. Under certain conditions, however, the "exchange of glasses" can lead to competition.

DRINKING COMPETITIONS: WHEN THE ROUND ACCELERATES

Under certain circumstances, the convivial exchange of drinks can accelerate, spiraling into a scene of collective, deliberate intoxication. Peppered with songs, jokes, and laughter, the invitation to drink cannot be refused, nor can it go unreturned. Excessive alcohol consumption in a group, particularly among male drinkers, then can become a performance by men standing, glasses raised, against the wind and the tides of the inner storms of drunkenness. Illustrations of such performances in literature, art, and, indeed, everyday life are countless (e.g., Nahoum-Grappe, 1991). The logic of the gift exchange at such drinking jousts goes beyond merely establishing a social connection within groups to include a struggle, however playful or tactical. Scenes from the 16th-century novels *The Histories of Gargantua and Pantagruel* by François Rabelais (1564/1955) offer glimpses into this world, where "he who does not feel the pleasure [i.e., intoxication] from alcohol drinks in vain." A 21st-century drinker would recognize the scenes of communal drunkenness described by Rabelais: the invitations to drink and the procession of raised glasses accompanying and setting the pace for a change in ambiance from the ordinary time of sobriety to the more exceptional time of drunkenness.

In writing about the world of thieves, Balzac (1838–1847/1997) described "orgies of strong liquors by which the triumph is celebrated" (p. 837). Around the Mediterranean, such group drinking customs have been depicted in great religious and literary texts since the ancient times. In *The Aeneid* by Virgil, for example, we find reciprocal drinking employed as a murderous tactic under the guise of celebratory drinking offered by women: "she spoke and poured an offering of wine onto the table and after the libation was the first to touch the bowl to her lips/Then she gave it to Bitias, challenging him: he briskly drained the brimming cup/drenching himself in its golden fullness." Bitias cannot refuse and does not detect the treachery behind the traditional act of friendship, the offer to drink.

From the joy of exchanging drinks under the rule of reciprocity, to a series of "swigs" in a group drinking to get drunk, to the tactical use of the intoxication of others to weaken opponents, the round as competition, coded or implicit, between men, usually warriors, is a recurring theme, particularly in the Old Regime France. Numerous texts of a literary as well as a religious or legal nature cite the act of making a toast as leading to a possible escalation of drinking, driven by ritual, politeness, and, among men, the drive to prove one's virility. The "winner" of the competitive round is not the one who refuses in the name of prudence or reason, but the one who risks the most and lasts the longest, commanding respect in the group and gaining authority over others, however temporary. This authority does not stem from physical strength or social success outside of the drinking context but, rather, is dependent on a display of power over oneself, revealed through excessive behavior.

Complex power play, thus, is often part of the practice of the round. A means to bond, a festive drinking scene can also give rise to a duel. The exchange of pleasantries between drinking companions follows a particular turn, like a battle, a joust of remarks—when laughter erupts, it means that an invisible target has been "hit." The funniest, the craziest, the most "radical" in the group becomes king for a night. Reciprocal drinking intensifies and escalates as the collective performance progresses, and a refusal of the next drink is taken as a sign of desertion. The drinker, particularly the male drinker, can jeopardize his established status and the basic foundation of his identity if he fails to keep up. Intoxication during the round can become a tactical weapon for "possessing" the other and, at the same time, a means of abandoning oneself, surrendering to stronger companions. What remains of the boisterous self, dancing on a thread, are the personal effects of a defrocked drunkard, in other words a skin, that physical part of the *I* deserted by the *self.*

Whatever the nature of the round, the drinking session revolves around the logic of reciprocity. As in war, you have to return "blows" received in a bar. This logic is rather masculine in its traditional version and attests to one of the functions of alcohol in modern society—a way to manipulate the atmosphere of a social gathering. The cordial offer of a drink to others is a sign of peace and alliance, but it also comes with an obligation to reciprocate, triggering a competition that can be a deliberate trap set for others, or for oneself.

CASE STUDY 3.2: Indigenous Australians and Alcohol

Creina Stockley and Anne Fox

Australia's indigenous peoples constitute only a small proportion (2.5%) of the overall population: According to the 2006 Census, 517,200 individuals identified as Aborigines or Torres Strait Islanders (Australian Bureau of Statistics, 2007). Of them, only approximately 24% still reside in traditionally oriented remote communities, and the rest live in mostly urban areas (see also Taylor, 2006). The median age of indigenous Australians is around 20 years (compared to about 36 years for their nonindigenous counterparts), with population growth constrained by high mortality: There is a 17-year difference in life expectancy between indigenous and nonindigenous groups.

In terms of alcohol consumption, indigenous communities report higher rates of both abstinence and heavy drinking than the general population (e.g., Hunter, 1992; Perkins et al., 1994); among those indigenous people who do drink, patterns, levels, and outcomes tend to be more harmful (Gray et al., 2000; Kelly, 2006). Overall, indigenous Australians exhibit higher than average rates of economic, health, and social problems, and there is no question that risky drinking contributes to ill health and premature mortality in this population. Two questions are at the heart of this case study: How did these problems arise, and what has been done about them?

HOW DID THE PROBLEMS ARISE?

To answer the first question, several theories have been proposed, pointing toward genetics, aftermath of colonization and cultural dislocation, Aboriginal experience with intoxicants prior to colonization, and drunkenness as protest against oppression.

Genetic Differences

It has been suggested that genetic variation in alcohol metabolism may explain the perceived Aboriginal vulnerability to alcohol effects, as has been observed in Chinese, Japanese, and Polynesian populations (Chambers et al., 2002; Dohmen et al., 1996; Shibuya & Yoshida, 1988; Thomasson et al., 1991; see also Chapter 2). However, the only study that examined this in Australians found no difference between indigenous and nonindigenous groups (Marinovich, Larsson, & Barber, 1976). So the most curious aspect of this argument is, as d'Abbs (2001a) put it, the "thirst for genetic explanations" in the Australian media. Hunter (1993) found that even proposed research on the subject was hailed in the media as an actual discovery of difference, citing some misleading headlines as examples (e.g., "Aborigines show alcohol problems may be genetic" and "One man's drink, another's poison") (p. 95). Several writers have commented that such myths can contribute to negative stereotyping and the development of so-called learned helplessness in Aboriginal people.

The confusion may have arisen because there *are* some genetic differences between indigenous and White Australians that can have a profound effect on lifestyle. Studies have found that indigenous groups from Australia (and Canada) are at higher than average risk of Type 2 diabetes. This is mainly the result of both a genetic predisposition and the adoption of unhealthy Westernized lifestyles. The body type and metabolism of Australian Aborigines are geared toward survival and fitness in the active life of a hunter-gatherer: For example, such features as mild glucose intolerance, relatively high cholesterol, and low body mass index enabled them to survive and gain weight on less food than would be necessary for European-descended Australians. Traditional hunter-gatherer diet would also have consisted of high-fiber, low-fat foods. Within the modern sedentary lifestyle and high-sugar, high-fat diet, however, such features become a drawback, resulting in widespread obesity and diabetes (Milton, 2000).

Aftermath of Colonization

The second most prevalent theory on the origin of harmful drinking among indigenous Australians focuses on the aftermath of European colonization. Problems seem to follow a classic pattern found in other displaced hunter-gatherer peoples, such as Native Americans in the United States, First Nations in Canada, and many African tribes (e.g., Akyeampong, 1996; Ishii, 2008). For most indigenous groups in the world, colonization has meant anything from cultural dislocation, prejudice, and stereotyping to extremes of political oppression, discrimination, violence, and slavery. Although the most racist and oppressive government actions have ceased, economic and educational disadvantages have resulted in poor health for many indigenous Australians (e.g., Couzos & Murray, 1999; Gray & Saggers, 1994). And, as illustrated by the following discussion, some would argue that certain forms of discrimination still continue under the guise of alcohol-management policies.

Alcohol was introduced to indigenous Australians by the British in 1788. Langton (1993) painted a depressing picture of this process:

> The image of the "drunken Aborigine" is a colonial construction which predated the ready availability of alcohol to Aboriginal people. From the first settlement and throughout the frontier period, alcohol was used to engage Aboriginal people in discourse, attract Aboriginal people into settlements, in barter for sexual favours from Aboriginal women, as payment for Aboriginal labour and to incite Aboriginal people to fight as street entertainment. Later, as the Aboriginal population was perceived to be a menace to further land dispossession, the protectionist policies involved a total ban on sale of alcohol to Aboriginal people, as well as opium in some regions, such as Queensland and the Northern Territory. (pp. 195–196)

Prohibitions against Aboriginal drinking were initiated in 1838, and by 1930, the licensing acts of all six Australian states and two territories included clauses prohibiting the sale of alcohol to indigenous groups (McKnight, 2002, p. 193). Although in some places, restrictions may have been imposed out of genuine concern for this population's welfare, in others they resulted from a fear of "uncontrollable intoxicated natives" (W. Brady, 2007). Some authors have argued that these bans have contributed to the rise of a heavy-drinking culture among indigenous groups (Elkin, 1958); others drew attention to the hypocrisy of these restrictions, citing evidence that extreme drinking was the norm among White Australians at the time and arguing that it was, in fact, this example that provided a template for Aboriginal drinking behavior (McKnight, 2002). In the 1800s, colonists, visitors, and missionaries described Australia as "a rum colony," and spoke of White settlers as being "completely lost in drink" (McKnight, 2002, p. 193). As Marshall (1979) concluded, "Peoples who lacked alcoholic beverages aboriginally borrowed styles of drunken comportment … from those who introduced them to the 'demon rum'" (p. 455). Although most Australian states had repealed full prohibition on alcohol sales to indigenous groups by 1965 (and, on reserves, by 1971), restrictive policies directed at this population's drinking continue to be enforced in many areas (McKnight, 2002). In some respects, as discussed later, these are implemented with the consent and cooperation of Aboriginal leaders, but in others the policies are strongly opposed.

As an explanation for Aboriginal drinking, the "aftereffects of colonization" theory has fallen out of favor in recent years as it is felt to be disempowering and potentially leading to a victim mentality. Unfortunately, this means that little research concentrates on aspects of indigenous drinking that may stem from, for example, cultural dislocation, discrimination, racism, and so on. Although there may be a recognizable grain of truth in it, the Australian government's explanation for the development of harmful drinking patterns among Aborigines is touchingly childlike in its storybook simplicity:

> Until about forty years ago [i.e., 1960s], Aboriginal and Torres Strait Islander peoples were not allowed to consume alcohol. If people wanted to drink, they would buy large quantities of alcohol and drink it quickly to avoid being caught and incarcerated. Such drinking often occurred in groups in the open air, on riverbanks and in parks. This was the genesis of patterns of drinking at harmful and hazardous levels. This pattern of drinking within the group afforded the people a sense of identity and belonging often denied as part of the colonisation process.

> Consuming alcohol in groups allowed people to be with family, receive news of other family members, to speak their language, sing songs, tell stories and pursue other activities. Consequently the sharing of alcohol, which is a part of wider cultural practice, had both positive and negative effects on the wellbeing of the Aboriginal and Torres Strait Islander people involved. The pattern of drinking large amounts in a short period of time has been handed down from one generation to the next. (Ministerial Council on Drug Strategy, 2006, p. 2)

Some nuance is added by work on drinking motives. Nichols (2002), for example, found that in her sample of Aborigines, lifetime abstainers tended to be those "who had the most opportunity to gain a sense of 'cultural knowing and belonging' in childhood, coupled with relative success in socio-economic terms" (p. 163). Economic success itself, however, in the absence of a strong sense of "Aboriginality" and knowledge of Aboriginal culture, was not associated with abstention or moderation—rather, the greatest numbers of current drinkers in the sample were found among those who were employed and had houses, cars, and other material comforts. Nichols concluded that "this is a possible indication, requiring far more exploration, that 'cultural'/psychological rather than economic impacts have played a greater role in [Aboriginal] people's past or present drinking decisions" (p. 164).

Prior Use of Intoxicants

Broome (1982/2002) suggested that Aborigines were "primed" for alcohol consumption by virtue of their previous knowledge of intoxicating substances. Their "craving" for alcohol, he suggested, "was no doubt rooted in their prior experience" (p. 58). For example, Stack (1989) elaborated on the preparation and traditional use of *pituri* (or *pitcheri*), dried fragments of the *Duboisia hopwoodii* plant mixed with wood ash and chewed in small quantities. This substance contains a form of nicotine that, although a stimulant, can also produce a pleasant intoxicating effect in moderate doses and hallucinations, coma, and even death in large doses.

> Within a few minutes of chewing it, a feeling of happy detachment results, with indifference to worry and physical hardship—the Aboriginal parallel to our use of alcohol. As a sustaining drug, it was vital to their long treks through the desert and semi-desert regions to

> deaden the cravings of hunger and for support with excessive fatigue. As a highly valued drug, the privilege of using it usually remained with the old men of the tribe who most jealously insisted that it was theirs alone. Women and young men did not normally enjoy *pituri*. In some tribes the old men, when faced with a serious undertaking such as a fight or a discussion of serious business, made sure that they masticated their quid of *pituri* first, chewing it from time to time and placing it behind the ear of the owner or that of the man next in line. … As nicotine is well known to spread via the trans-dermal route, then the absorption of the drug continued while resting behind the ear. … Its use is also thought to play a major part in promoting altered consciousness in initiation rites and other special rituals. With heavy use, its ability to produce hallucinations would certainly enhance the mystic power of the initiation rite. (p. 4)

This implies that, like many other indigenous peoples, Australian Aborigines have historically developed cultural practices to regulate the use of intoxicating substances, so their modern problems cannot stem from a lack of capability in this regard.

However, it appears to be a universal human phenomenon that such cultural practices tend to be substance-specific: Social rules and regulations that control the use of one substance are not necessarily transferable to another, and, when the core binding elements of a culture are torn apart by loss of habitat, political oppression, enslavement, genocide, or other negative forces, there is little chance for social regulation to develop about a new substance. Drunken comportment, as anthropologists have found the world over, is a *learned* behavior: Like McKnight (2002) and others have suggested, Australian Aborigines can only have learned it from White settlers.

Drunkenness as Protest

Several anthropologists have observed that drunken behavior may constitute political rebellion and a statement of sovereignty of the physical self. In a U.S. study, Olson and Wilson (1985), for example, described the outcomes of disappearance on Native American reservations of opportunities for "public confirmations of Indian-ness":

> Some Native Americans institutionalized drunkenness as a form of protest against the dominant society. Among loosely organized tribes occupying unfamiliar reservations, public drunkenness was more

> common. … By becoming publicly drunk, they purposefully fulfilled the stereotype [of the drunken Indian], confirming to themselves and to others that they really were Native Americans and were not ashamed of it. (p. 54)

Hutchings (1993) and others applied this theory to indigenous Australians:

> Self-destruction of the body through the use of drugs and alcohol and self-mutilation are the ultimate statements of resistance. To "run amok" is to construct the self as disordered in the face of a system attempting to impose order and authority over Aboriginal children's lives. In doing this, Aboriginal children introduce some disorder to the system at the ground level. More than this, self-abuse of the body is an attempt to retain self identity and direction over one's destiny by defining the body as the locus over which outside forces have limited control, but which the individual has the power to destroy. (p. 358)

WHAT HAS BEEN DONE?

Australian government responses have been varied. The 2006–2009 Alcohol Strategy had little to say about indigenous drinking, aside from highlighting two interventions for which it claimed success, the Living with Alcohol program (LWAP) and the sobering-up centers. These two initiatives are worth reviewing as examples of what has been done.

Living With Alcohol Program

The government of the Northern Territory (where indigenous peoples make up 31.6% of the population, the largest indigenous presence in percentage terms among Australian states and territories) implemented LWAP from 1992 to 2000. The program included both general and community-based initiatives and was thought to be culturally relevant for indigenous communities, as they were involved in some elements of its design and delivery. LWAP aimed to bring the level of alcohol consumption and related harm in the Northern Territory and its remote communities down to national levels by 2002. It used strategies such as increased controls on alcohol availability and expanded education, drink-driver programs, night-patrol initiatives, rehabilitation and treatment facilities, and other services (d'Abbs, 2001a, 2004;

Stockwell et al., 2001). From 1992 to 1997, LWAP was funded by state levy on sales of drinks with alcohol content above 3% ABV.

At the community level, the program's emphasis was on local alcohol availability restrictions, focusing in particular on takeaway sales of cask wine. Many jurisdictions placed limits or bans on, for example, admission of children to public bars, third-party sales (e.g., to taxi drivers), hours and days (e.g., Sundays and traditional paydays) of sale, and maximum purchase allowances. Bans on all alcohol sales to native Australians were implemented on some Ngaanyatjarra, Pitjantjatjara, and Yankunytjatjara (NPY) indigenous lands.

In the NPY, however, the Aboriginal people in the region of Curtin Springs, the Anangu, despite receiving funding to join LWAP, rejected the proposal after they were denied the right to self-administer it—the Northern Territory Liquor Commission insisted on retaining control. After several alcohol-related deaths and numerous incidents of harm among Anangu drinkers, NPY leaders appealed in July 1996 to the Race Discrimination Commission, requesting a Special Measures Application under section 8(1) of the Racial Discrimination Act (RDA) 1975 to apply to Curtin Springs, ensuring that the ban would not constitute a violation of human rights. This was eventually awarded, and the licensees were forced to stop selling almost all forms of alcohol to indigenous residents of the area (Australasian Legal Information Institute, 1999).

Evaluations of many LWAP elements found only modest impact on alcohol consumption, but some areas did demonstrate significant reductions in indicators of harm, especially criminal charges, violence, and alcohol-related road crashes (d'Abbs & Togni, 2000). For example, the Tennant Creek community, which called its LWAP initiative Beat the Grog, reported a 34% reduction in admissions to the accident and emergency department in connection with the initiative, citing decreases in general injuries, fractures, head injuries, gastrointestinal conditions, lacerations, and stab injuries (Gray, Saggers, Atkinson, Sputore, & Bourbon, 2000). These results were sustained over the life of LWAP so that alcohol-related harm was reduced both in the short and long term in the Northern Territory (Chikritzhs, Stockwell, & Pascal, 2005; Stockwell et al., 2001).

The evaluators' conclusions, however, were not unequivocal. At least three confounding factors were identified (Chikritzhs, Stockwell, Pascal, & Catalano, 2004):

1. Per capita alcohol consumption was already on a clear downward trend when LWAP was introduced and may have continued its course without the program.
2. Declines in acute alcohol-attributable deaths in the Northern Territory occurred about 1 year before the official implementation of LWAP.
3. The period of the program's evaluation coincided with an economic recession, which, historically, has also been associated with reductions in per-capita alcohol consumption.

As Stockwell et al. (2001) concluded, "The extent to which these benefits can be entirely attributed to the [LWAP] levy, the programmes funded by [LWAP], or other initiatives or changes in economic activity is unclear" (pp. 178–179).

In some areas, government projects such as LWAP received widespread support in indigenous communities; other programs, however, have been labeled racist, sparking protests among Aborigines. For example, protesters marched on Canberra in 2007 after the government took control of welfare payments, issuing food credits instead of cash to stop indigenous people from purchasing alcohol. Although many local NPY authorities actively sought to impose an alcohol sales ban on their own people, some indigenous residents have vociferously opposed these measures implemented under section 8 of the RDA. For example, the Palm Island Aboriginal Shire Council (PIASC) unanimously agreed that the State Government's Alcohol Management Plan (AMP) was "heavy-handed" and "racist," criminalizing people and applying "outrageous" fines for "simply having a drink." To qualify for a section 8, an AMP must have the support of the community, which the Palm Island AMP clearly did not. The issues paper prepared by the PIASC cited many objections, including a lack of consultation and negotiation with local people and a gross misapplication of government money. The funding for the AMP, the PIASC claimed, included no provision for desperately needed support projects such as rehabilitation centers.

D'Abbs (2001b) concluded that the inclusion of "social controls" (composed of both informal social controls, "based on values and understandings sustained within lifeworlds," and formal agencies, such as licensing authorities and the police) in models of harm reduction would make initiatives more culturally relevant to Aborigines (p. 49). The preceding examples demonstrate that indigenous communities in Australia have differing needs and attitudes in terms of alcohol policy. For many areas, strong elements of formal alcohol control are indeed welcomed, but most want the right to administer their own programs and regulations.

Sobering-Up Centers

Another community-based initiative provides sobering-up centers, established across Australia. These facilities offer safe overnight accommodation for publicly intoxicated individuals (who have committed no criminal offense) as an alternative to arrest and police detention. The first sobering-up center opened in Darwin, Northern Territory, in 1983. Public drunkenness was decriminalized in the Northern Territory in 1974, but alternative care was not mandated (as it was done, e.g., in New South Wales) for another 7 years, during which time significant numbers of indigenous Australians were apprehended and held in police custody without being charged. For example, in the city of Darwin between 1974 and 1982, a 106% increase in the number of persons taken into custody for being drunk was reported, suggesting that the policy was "decriminalisation in name only" (Donald, 1984). In 1983, 94% of protective custody apprehensions in another Northern Territory town, Tennant Creek, were of indigenous Australians (M. Brady, 1988).

The Royal Commission into Aboriginal Deaths in Custody facilitated the establishment of sobering-up centers across the country in response to this situation, looking to prevent negative outcomes of police involvement in public drunkenness and minimize alcohol-related injury in Aboriginal people. In the state of South Australia, 6,486 admissions to such centers were recorded between 1991 and 2000; indigenous Australians accounted for 97.1% of these cases (M. Brady, Nicholls, Henderson, & Byrne, 2006). Researchers linked the high prevalence of indigenous people to the extent of their public drinking, a lack of appropriate accommodation, the role of the town as a service hub for indigenous communities in the broader region, and the activities of Mobile Assistance Patrols (MAPs) initiated by the Aboriginal Sobriety Group (M. Brady et al., 2006; Byrne, Brady, & Henderson, 2001). Large numbers of indigenous Australians travel through the region in association with periodic ceremonial activity and as part of the normative high mobility of desert people (Peterson, 2004; Taylor & Bell, 2004).

Sobering-up centers help reduce social disruption and violence by and against drunk individuals in public areas, and lower costs of health and law enforcement agencies. They are not treatment facilities but can identify and refer customers to appropriate health care services. Although no formal evaluation of the centers has been conducted, no accident or complaint has been recorded at a center to date.

Although the sobering-up facilities and the MAPs are generally viewed as far more helpful than police response (and, because MAPs are staffed by indigenous Australians, as more culturally sensitive), government policies aimed to reduce public drunkenness and their enforcement have been accused of unfairly targeting itinerant or homeless Aboriginal people (Blagg & Valuri, 2003). As William Jonas, the Race Discrimination Commissioner, observed:

> The trend has continued of State and local governments resurrecting old policies of segregating and excluding Aboriginal people from public places. These laws and policies in theory apply to everyone, but in practice target Aboriginal people. … They are based on paternalistic notions about the relationship between government and Indigenous people and attempt to impose assimilation as a pre-condition to their acceptance as full members of society. They come close to violating the citizenship rights of Aboriginal people. They also ignore the history of Aboriginal exclusion and disadvantage. They impact on the poorest, most isolated and most disadvantaged. Aboriginal people are grossly over-represented among those afflicted by ill-health (including alcohol addiction), poor living conditions and homelessness. It is frankly disingenuous to claim that such laws target behaviour pure and simple, without any racial component. (pp. 148, 149–150)

Critics have drawn attention to the cultural significance to Aboriginal people of many public spaces, places where communities get together (and sometimes drink alcohol). Hall (2004), for example, has chronicled the history of Adelaide's public spaces: In the post–World War II era,

> the City Squares of Adelaide were to become an important venue for Indigenous sociality and solidarity. In the most public of City spaces Indigenous people were able to enjoy the intimacy of family and friends and assert for themselves a place and identity within the City. Indigenous sociality played out in the City's heartland did not however enjoy the approbation of the wider community. Rather it was to become subject to intensified surveillance and official attempts at control. (p. 56)

In a report on the cultural significance of the parks, Hemming (1998) cited the following statement from the Kaurna people in South Australia:

> The setting-up of the City of Adelaide and its Park Lands deprived our ancestors of the responsibility for maintaining crucial, culturally meaningful places. On the Park Lands the Kaurna have suffered to the present day as a result of this dispossession. Invasion has meant continuing alienation, oppression and harassment for us and other indigenous people. These injustices have been planted out on the Adelaide Park Lands. The Park Lands have many culturally significant places. These places should be preserved from further encroachment. We, as Kaurna people, must walk on these places to maintain our cultural strength. (p. 16)

CONCLUSION

Anthropological concerns about the origins of cultural problems can seem irrelevant in the face of real modern-day problems, and many would rightly argue that a return to traditional bush life is neither realistic nor desirable for many indigenous Australians, but, without an understanding of the causes of drunkenness, solutions to these public problems, although often well meaning, are usually misguided and ineffective. Cultural problems need cultural solutions. A deeper understanding of the social and cultural losses that the indigenous communities have suffered could lead to more appropriate rehabilitative programs and social policy. From the evidence set out here, it is apparent that Aboriginal drinking can only be curbed through genuine empowerment and self-determination.

REFERENCES

Adams, D. (2004). *The hitchhiker's guide to the galaxy.* London: Harmony. (Original work published 1979)

Akyeampong, E. (1996). *Drink, power, and cultural change: A social history of alcohol in Ghana, c. 1800 to recent times.* Portsmouth, NH: Heineman.

Alexander, B. K. (2001, January 21). *The myth of drug-induced addiction.* Paper delivered to the Canadian Senate. Retrieved December 12, 2009, from http://www.parl.gc.ca/37/1/parlbus/commbus/senate/Com-e/ille-e/presentation-e/alexender-e.htm

Assefi, S. L., & Garry, M. (2003). Absolut memory distortions: Alcohol placebos influence the misinformation effect. *Psychological Science, 14,* 77–80.

Australasian Legal Information Institute. (1999). Curtin Springs roadhouse: Ten years of community struggle. *Indigenous Law Bulletin* [Online]. Retrieved October 20, 2009, from http://www.austlii.edu.au/au/journals/ILB/1999/24.html

Australian Bureau of Statistics. (2007). *Population distribution, Aboriginal and Torres Strait Islander Australians, 2006.* Retrieved November 30, 2009, from http://www.abs.gov.au

Balzac, H. (1997). *Splendeur et misère des courtisanes* [The splendors and miseries of courtesans]. Paris: Editions Flammarion. (Original work published 1838–1847)

Barkow, H. J., Cosmides, L., & Tooby, J. (Eds.). (1992). *The adapted mind: Evolutionary psychology and the generation of culture.* Oxford, UK: Oxford University Press.

Barrett, L., Dunbar, R., & Lycett, J. (2001). *Human evolutionary psychology.* Basingstoke, UK: Palgrave Macmillan.

Blagg, H., & Valuri, G. (2003). *An overview of night patrol services in Australia.* Canberra, Australia: Crime Prevention Branch, Commonwealth Attorney-General's Department.

Boyd, R., & Richerson, P. J. (2005). *The origin and evolution of cultures.* Oxford, UK: Oxford University Press.

Bradley, M. T., & Ainsworth, D. (1984). Alcohol and psychophysiological detection of deception. *Psychophysiology, 21,* 63–67.

Brady, M. (1988). *Where the beer truck stopped: Drinking in a northern Australian town.* Darwin, Australia: Australian National University, North Australia Research Unit.

Brady, M., Nicholls, R., Henderson, G., & Byrne, J. (2006). The role of a rural sobering-up centre in managing alcohol-related harm to Aboriginal people in South Australia. *Drug and Alcohol Review, 25,* 201–206.

Brady, W. (2007). The sovereign being: History matters. In A. Moreton-Robinson (Ed.), *Sovereign subjects: Indigenous sovereignty matters* (pp. 140–153). Crows Nest, Australia: Allen & Unwin.

Braidwood, R. J., Sauer, J. D., Helbaek, H., Mangelsdorf, P. C., Cutler, H. C., Coon, C. S., et al. (1953). Symposium: Did man once live by beer alone? *American Anthropologist, 55,* 515–526.

Broome, R. (2002). *Aboriginal Australians.* Crows Nest, Australia: Allen & Unwin. (Original work published 1982)

Brown, W. M., & Moore, C. (2000). Is prospective altruist-detection an evolved solution to the adaptive problem of subtle cheating in cooperative ventures? Supportive evidence using the Wason selection task. *Evolution and Human Behavior, 21,* 25–37.

Butler, B. Y. (2006). *Holy intoxication to drunken dissipation: Alcohol among Quichua speakers in Otavalo, Ecuador.* Albuquerque: University of New Mexico Press.

Byrne, J., Brady, M., & Henderson, G. (2001). *Monitoring the long-term social and environmental effects of changes in alcohol availability in an Aboriginal community: A ten-year follow up study.* Unpublished report, Yalata Community. South Australia.

Campbell, M. A. (1991). Public drinking places and society. In D. J. Pittman & H. R. White (Eds.), *Society, culture and drinking patterns reexamined* (pp. 361–380). New Brunswick, NJ: Rutgers Center for Alcohol Studies.

Chambers, G. K., Marshall, S. J., Robinson, G. M., Maguire, S., Newton-Howes, J., & Chong, N. L. (2002). Genetics of alcoholism in Polynesians: Alcohol and aldehyde dehydrogenase genotypes in young men. *Alcoholism: Clinical and Experimental Research, 26,* 949–955.

Chikritzhs, T., Stockwell, T., & Pascal, R. (2005). The impact of the Northern Territory's Living with Alcohol program, 1992–2002: Revisiting the evaluation. *Addiction, 100,* 1625–1636.

Chikritzhs, T. N., Stockwell, T. R., Pascal, R., & Catalano, P. (2004). *The Northern Territory's Living with Alcohol program, 1992–2002: Revisiting the evaluation.* Perth, Australia: National Drug Research Institute, Curtin University of Technology.

Cohen, M. N., & Armelagos, G. J. (Eds.). (1984). *Paleopathology at the origins of agriculture.* Orlando, FL: Academic Press.

Cosmides, L., & Tooby, J. (1992). Cognitive adaptations for social exchange. In H. J. Barkow, L. Cosmides, & J. Tooby (Eds.), *The adapted mind: Evolutionary psychology and the generation of culture* (pp. 163–228). Oxford, UK: Oxford University Press.

Couzos, S., & Murray, R. (1999). *Aboriginal primary health care: An evidence-based approach.* Melbourne, Australia: Oxford University Press.

Cunliffe, B. (1988). *Greeks, Romans and Barbarians: Spheres of interaction.* Swindon, UK: Book Club Associates.

d'Abbs, P. (2001a). Living with Alcohol: Learning from the Northern Territory experience. *Drug and Alcohol Review, 20,* 253–255.

d'Abbs, P. (2001b). Silence of the sociologists: Indigenous alcohol use, harm minimisation and social control. *Health Sociology Review, 10,* 33–52.

d'Abbs, P. (2004). Alignment of the policy planets: Behind the implementation of the Northern Territory (Australia) Living with Alcohol program. *Drug and Alcohol Review, 23,* 55–65.

d'Abbs, P., & Togni, S. (2000). Liquor licensing and community action in regional and remote Australia: Review of recent initiatives. *Australian and New Zealand Journal of Public Health, 24,* 45–53.

Dennis, P. A. (1979). The role of the drunk in an Oaxacan village. In M. Marshall (Ed.), *Beliefs, behaviors and alcoholic beverages* (pp. 54–64). Ann Arbor: University of Michigan Press.

Dohmen, K., Baraona, E., Ishibashi, H., Pozzato, G., Moretti, M., Matsunaga, C., et al. (1996). Ethnic differences in gastric sigma-alcohol dehydrogenase activity and ethanol first-pass metabolism. *Alcoholism: Clinical and Experimental Research, 20,* 1569–1576.

de Garine, I., & de Garine, V. (Eds.). (2001). *Drinking: Anthropological approaches.* New York: Berghahn Books.

de Rojas, J. L. (1998). El calendario festivo azteca [The Aztec festive calendar]. In H. Perez Martinez (Ed.), *Mexico en fiesta* (pp. 241–254). Zamora, Mexico: El Colegio de Michoacan.

Descombes, V. (1996). *Les institutions du sens* [Institutions of meaning]. Paris: Editions de minuit.

Diamond, J. M. (2004). *The third chimpanzee: The evolution and future of the human animal.* Santa Fe, NM: Radius. (Original work published 1991 as *The rise and fall of the third chimpanzee: How our animal heritage affects the way we live*)

Donald, W. (1984). *Public drunkenness: Decriminalization and the exercise of police discretion in the Northern Territory.* Honors thesis, Australian National University, Canberra, Australia.

Douglas, M. (Ed.). (1987). *Constructive drinking: Perspectives on drink from anthropology.* London: Routledge.

Dudley, R. (2000). Evolutionary origins of human alcoholism in primate frugivory. *Quarterly Review of Biology, 75,* 3–15.

Dudley, R. (2002). Fermenting fruit and the historical ecology of ethanol ingestion: Is alcoholism in modern humans an evolutionary hangover? *Addiction, 97,* 381–388.

Dunbar, R. (1997). *Grooming, gossip and the evolution of language.* Cambridge, MA: Harvard University Press.

Durkheim, E. (2008). *The elementary forms of the religious life* (K. E. Fields, Trans.). Oxford, UK: Oxford Paperbacks. (Original work published 1912)

Edwards, G. (2000). *Alcohol: The world's favorite drug.* New York: St. Martin's.

Ehrlich, P. R. (2000). *Human natures: Genes, cultures and the human prospect.* Washington, DC: Island Press.

Elkin, A. P. (1958). *Aborigines and citizenship.* Sydney: Association for the Protection of Native Races.

Engs, R. C. (1995). Do traditional western European drinking practices have origins in antiquity? *Addiction Research, 2,* 227–239.

Fakjær, H. O. (1992). *Alkohol og narkotika myter og virkelighet* [The psychology of getting high]. Oslo, Norway: Gyldendal.

Fillmore, M. T., & Vogel-Sprott, M. (2000). Response inhibition under alcohol: Effects of cognitive and motivational conflict. *Journal of Studies on Alcohol, 61,* 239–246.

Fox, A. (2007, October). *Cultural perspective.* Speech at the Workshop on Intoxication and Drunkenness of the International Center for Alcohol Policies and DrinkWise Australia, Paris.

Fox, A. (in press). *Drink and duty: Drinking culture in the British Army.* Unpublished doctoral dissertation, Imperial College London.

Fox, K. (1999). *Social and cultural aspects of drinking.* London: Amsterdam Group

Fox, K. (2004). *Evolution, alienation and gossip: The role of mobile telecommunications in the 21st century.* Oxford, UK: Social Issues Research Centre (SIRC). Retrieved September 10, 2009, from http://www.sirc.org/publik/gossip.shtml

Fox, K. (2008). *Watching the English: The hidden rules of English behaviour.* London: Nicholas Brealey.

Fox, R. (1991). *Encounter with anthropology.* New Brunswick, NJ: Transaction Publishers.

Fox, R. (2000). *The passionate mind: Sources of destruction and creativity.* New Brunswick, NJ: Transaction.

Fox, R. (in press). *The tribal imagination: Civilization and the savage mind.* Cambridge, MA: Harvard University Press.

Geller, I. (1971). Ethanol preference in rats as a function of photoperiod. *Science, 173,* 456–458.

George, W. H., & Norris, J. (1991). Alcohol, disinhibition, sexual arousal, and deviant sexual behaviour. *Alcohol Health and Research World, 15,* 133–138.

Giancola, P. R. (2002a). Alcohol-related aggression during the college years: Theories, risk factors and policy implications. *Journal of Studies on Alcohol, 14*(Suppl.), 129–139.

Giancola, P. R. (2002b). Alcohol-related aggression in men and women: The influence of dispositional aggressivity. *Journal of Studies on Alcohol, 63,* 696–708.

Giancola, P. R., Helton, E. L., Osborne, A. B., Terry, M. K., Fuss, A. M., & Westerfield, J. A. (2002). The effects of alcohol and provocation on aggressive behavior in men and women. *Journal of Studies on Alcohol, 63,* 64–73.

Gilman, J. M., Ramchandani, V. A., Davis, M. B., Bjork, J. M., & Hommer, D. W. (2008). Why we like to drink: A functional magnetic resonance imaging study of the rewarding and anxiolytic effects of alcohol. *The Journal of Neuroscience, 28,* 4583–4591.

Godelier, M. (1996). *L'Enigme du don* [The enigma of the gift]. Paris: Grasset.

Goffman, E. (1974). Perdre la face ou faire bonne figure [To lose face or to make a good impression]. In E. Goffman (Ed.), *Les rites d'interaction* (pp. 7–42). Paris: Les éditions de minuit.

Goffman, E. (1975). *Mise en scène de la vie quotidienne* [The presentation of self in everyday life]. Paris: Les éditions de minuit.

Gray, D., & Saggers, S. (1994). Aboriginal health: The harvest of injustice. In C. Waddell & A. Petersen (Eds.), *Just health* (pp. 119–133). Melbourne, Australia: Churchill Livingstone.

Gray, D., Saggers, S., Atkinson, D., Sputore, B., & Bourbon, D. (2000). Beating the grog: Evaluation of the Tennant Creek liquor licensing restrictions. *Australian and New Zealand Journal of Public Health, 24,* 39–44.

Gusfield, J. R. (1996). *Contested meanings: The construction of alcohol problems.* Madison, WI: University of Wisconsin Press.

Hajar, R. (2000). Alcohol: Friend or foe? A historical perspective. *Heart Views, 1,* 341–344.

Hall, L.-A. (2004). Sitting down in the square: Indigenous in an Australian city. *Humanities Research, 11,* 54–77.

Harlan, J. R. (1967). A wild wheat harvest in Turkey. *Archaeology, 20,* 197–201.

Hecht, J. (2008, 28 July). Boozy tree shrews avoid fermented hangovers. *New Scientist* [Online]. Retrieved September 30, 2009, from http://www.newscientist.com/article/dn14411-boozy-tree-shrews-avoid-fermented-fruit-hangovers.html

Hemming, S. (1998). *A report on the indigenous cultural significance of the Adelaide park lands.* Adelaide, Australia: Adelaide City Council.

Hornsey, I. S. (2003). *A history of beer and brewing.* Cambridge, UK: Royal Academy of Chemistry.

Hunter, E. (1992). Aboriginal alcohol use: A review of quantitative studies. *Journal of Drug Issues, 22,* 713–731.

Hunter, E. (1993). *Aboriginal health and history: Power and prejudice in remote Australia.* Cambridge, UK: Cambridge University Press.

Hutchings, S. (1993). The great shoe store robbery. *Oceania, 63,* 345–362.

Ishii, I. (2008). *Bad fruits of the civilized tree: Alcohol and the sovereignty of the Cherokee nation.* Lincoln: University of Nebraska Press.

Katz, S. H., & Voigt, M. M. (1987). Bread and beer: The early use of cereals in the human diet. *Expedition, 28,* 23–34.

Kelly, A. B. (2006). Alcohol problems and psychological health in a remote Indigenous Australian community: A preliminary quantitative study. *Australian Journal of Rural Health, 14,* 86–87.

Kline, A. S. (2002). *Virgil: The Aeneid. Book I.* Retrieved on May 10, 2010, from http://www.poetryintranslation.com

Knight, C. (1990). *Blood relations: Menstruation and the origins of culture.* New Haven, CT: Yale University Press.

Kovacs, M. G. (1989). *The epic of Gilgamesh.* Palo Alto, CA: Stanford University Press.

Kuntsche, E., Rehm, J., & Gmel, G. (2004). Characteristics of binge drinkers in Europe. *Social Science and Medicine, 59,* 113–127.

Kuper, A. (1999). *Culture: The anthropologists' account.* Cambridge, MA: Harvard University Press.

Langton, M. (1993). Rum, seduction and death: "Aboriginality" and alcohol. *Oceania, 63,* 195–207.

Levine, H. G. (1992). Temperance cultures: Alcohol as a problem in Nordic and English-speaking cultures. In M. Lader, G. Edwards, & C. Drummond (Eds.), *The nature of alcohol and drug-related problems* (pp. 15–36). Oxford, UK: Oxford University Press.

Lévi-Strauss, C. (1967). *Les structures élémentaires de la parenté* [The elementary structures of kinship]. Paris: Mouton.

Lewis-Williams, D., & Pearce, D. (2005). *Inside the Neolithic mind.* London: Thames & Hudson.

Mace, R., Holden, C. J., & Shennan, S. (Eds.). (2005). *The evolution of cultural diversity.* London: UCL Press.

Mandelbaum, D. G. (1965). Alcohol and culture. *Current Anthropology, 6,* 281–293.

Marinovich, N., Larsson, O., & Barber, K. (1976). Comparative metabolism rates of ethanol in adults of Aboriginal and European descent. *Medical Journal of Australia, 1*(Suppl.), 44–46.

Marshall, M. (1979). *Weekend warriors: Alcohol in a Micronesian culture (Explorations in world ethnology).* Mountain View, CA: Mayfield.

Mauss, M. (1923–1924). Essai sur le don: Forme et raison de l'échange dans les sociétés archaïques [An essay on the gift: The form and reason of exchange in archaic societies]. *L'Année Sociologique, 2.* Retrieved September 20, 2009, from http://classiques.uqac.ca/classiques/mauss_marcel/socio_et_anthropo/2_essai_sur_le_don/essai_sur_le_don.pdf

McDonald, M. (1994). *Gender, drink and drugs.* Oxford, UK: Berg.

McKnight, D. (2002). *From hunting to drinking: The devastating effects of alcohol on an Australian Aboriginal community.* London: Routledge.

Miczek, K. A., Hubbard, N., & Cantuti-Castelvetri, I. (1995). Increased cocaine self-administration after social stress. *Neuroscience Abstracts, 21,* 1954.

Milton, K. (2000). Hunter-gatherer diets—A different perspective. *American Journal of Clinical Nutrition, 71,* 665–667.

Ministerial Council on Drug Strategy. (2006, May). *National drug strategy: Aboriginal and Torres Strait Islander peoples complementary action plan 2003–2009. Background paper.* Canberra, Australia: National Drug Strategy Unit.

Mitchell, T. (2004). *Intoxicated identities: Alcohol's power in Mexican history and culture.* New York: Routledge.

Mithen, S. (1996). *The prehistory of the mind.* London: Thames and Hudson.

Morris, D. (2004). *The nature of happiness.* London: Little Book.

Nahoum-Grappe, V. (Ed.). (1991). *La culture de l'ivresse: Un essai de phénoménologie historique* [The culture of drunkenness: An essay on an historical phenomenon]. Paris: Quai Voltaire.

Nahoum-Grappe, V., Tsykounas, M., & Fillaut, T. (Eds.). (1998). *Histoire et alcool* [History and alcohol] (Vol. 2). Paris: L'Harmattan.

Nichols, F. T. (2002). *Identity, opportunity and hope: An Aboriginal model for alcohol (and other drug) harm prevention and intervention.* Unpublished doctoral dissertation, Curtin University of Technology, National Drug Research Institute, Australia.

Olson, J. S., & Wilson, R. (1985). *Native Americans in the twentieth century.* Chicago: University of Illinois Press.

Panter-Brick, C., Layton, R., & Rowley-Conwy, P. (Eds.). (2001). *Hunter-gatherers: An interdisciplinary perspective.* Cambridge, UK: Cambridge University Press.

Parker, L. L., Penton-Voak, I. S., Attwood, A. S., & Munafo, M. R. (2008). Effects of acute alcohol consumption on ratings of attractiveness of facial stimuli: Evidence of long-term encoding. *Alcohol and Alcoholism, 43,* 636–640.

Perkins, J. J., Sanson-Fisher, R. W., Blunden, S., Lunnay, D., Redman, S., & Hensley, M. J. (1994). Prevalence of drug use in urban Aboriginal communities. *Addiction, 89,* 1319–1331.

Peterson, N. (2004). Myth of the "walkabout": Movement in the Aboriginal domain. In J. Taylor & M. Bell (Eds.), *Population mobility and indigenous peoples in Australia and North America* (pp. 223–238). London: Routledge.

Pierson, D. S. (1999). Natural killers—Turning the tide of battle. *Military Review, 79,* 60–65.

Profet, M. (1992). Pregnancy sickness as adaptation: A deterrent to maternal ingestion of teratogens. In J. H. Barkow, L. Cosmides, & J. Tooby (Eds.), *The adapted mind: Evolutionary psychology and the generation of culture* (pp. 327–365). Oxford, UK: Oxford University Press.

Purcell, N. (1985). Wine and wealth in ancient Italy. *Journal of Roman Studies, 75,* 1–19

Rabelais, F. (1955). *The histories of Gargantua and Pantagruel* (J. M. Cohen, Trans.). New York: Penguin. (Original work published 1564)

Raitasalo, K., Knibbe, R., & Kraus, L. (2005). Retrieval strategies and cultural differences in answering survey questions on drinking: A cross-national comparison. *Addiction Research & Theory, 13,* 359–372.

Rehfisch, F. (2003). Competitive beer drinking among the Mambila. In M. Douglas (Ed.), *Constructive drinking: Perspectives on drink from anthropology* (pp. 135–145). London: Routledge. (Original work published 1987)

Room, R. (1980, August). *Alcohol as an instrument of intimate domination.* Paper presented at the annual meeting of the Society for the Studies of Social Problems, New York.

Room, R., & Mäkelä, K. (2000). Typologies of the cultural position of drinking. *Journal of Studies on Alcohol, 61,* 475–483.

Rooney, J. F. (1991). Patterns of alcohol use in Spanish society. In D. J. Pittman & H. R. White (Eds.), *Society, culture and drinking patterns re-examined: Alcohol, culture, and social control* (pp. 381–397). New Brunswick, NJ: Rutgers Center for Alcohol Studies.

Rousseau, J.-J. (1968). *The social contract* (M. Cranson, Trans.). London: Penguin. (Original work published 1762)

Rudgely, K. (1993). *The alchemy of culture: Intoxicants in society.* London: British Museum Press.

Rudgely, K. (1994). *Essential substances: A cultural history of intoxicants in society.* New York: Kodansha Globe.

Sherratt, A. (1991). Sacred and profane substances: The ritual use of narcotics in later Neolithic Europe. In P. Garwood, D. Jennings, R. Skeates, & J. Toms (Eds.), *Sacred and profane: Proceedings of a conference on archaeology, ritual and religion* (pp. 50–64). Oxford, UK: Oxford University Committee for Archaeology.

Shibuya, A., & Yoshida, A. (1988). Genotypes of alcohol-metabolizing enzymes in Japanese with alcohol liver diseases: A strong association of the usual Caucasian-type aldehyde dehydrogenase gene (ALDH super1/sub2). *American Journal of Human Genetics, 43,* 744–748.

Siegel, R. K. (1989). *Intoxication: Life in pursuit of artificial paradise.* London: Simon & Schuster.

Siegel, R. K. (2005). *Intoxication: The universal drive for mind-altering substances.* South Paris, ME: Park Street Press.

Southwick, L., Steele, C., Marlatt, A., & Lindell, M. (1981). Alcohol-related expectancies: Defined by phase of intoxication and drinking experience. *Journal of Consulting and Clinical Psychology, 49,* 713–772.

Stack, E. (1989). *Aboriginal pharmacopoeia* (Occasional Papers No. 10). Darwin, Australia: Northern Territory Library Service.

Steele, C. M., & Josephs, R. A. (1990). Alcohol myopia: Its prized and dangerous effects. *American Psychologist, 45,* 921–933.

Stockwell, T., Chikritzhs, T., Hendrie, D., Fordham, R., Ying, F., Phillips, M., et al. (2001). Public health and safety benefits of the Northern Territory's Living with Alcohol programme. *Drug and Alcohol Review, 20,* 167–180.

Stringer, C., & Andrews, P. (2005). *The complete world of human evolution.* London: Thames and Hudson.

Tanaka, T. (1980). *The San, hunter-gatherers of the Kalahari.* Tokyo, Japan: University of Tokyo Press.

Taylor, J. (2006). *Population and diversity: Policy implications of emerging Indigenous demographic trends* (CAEPR Discussion Paper No. 283). Canberra, Australia: Centre for Aboriginal Economic Policy Research, Australian National University.

Taylor, J., & Bell, M. (Eds.). (2004). *Population mobility and indigenous peoples in Australia and North America.* London: Routledge.

Thomasson, H. R., Edenberg, H. J., Crabb, D. W., Mai, X. L., Jerome, R. E., Li, T. K., et al. (1991). Alcohol and aldehyde dehydrogenase genotypes and alcoholism in Chinese men. *American Journal of Human Genetics, 48,* 677–681.

Trivers, R. (1971). The evolution of reciprocal altruism. *Quarterly Review of Biology, 46,* 35–57.

Turmo, I. G. (2001). Drinking: An almost silent language. In I. de Garine & V. de Garine (Eds.), *Drinking: Anthropological approaches* (pp. 130–143). New York: Berghahn Books.

Turner, V. (1995). *The ritual process: Structure and anti-structure.* Edison, NJ: Transaction. (Original work published 1969)

Vengeliene, V., Siegmund, S., Singer, M. V., Sinclair, J. D., Li, T. K., & Spanagel, R. (2003). A comparative study on alcohol-preferring rat lines: Effects of deprivation and stress phases on voluntary alcohol intake. *Alcoholism: Clinical and Experimental Research, 27,* 1048–1054.

Warburton, D. M. (1999). Pleasure for health. In S. Peele & M. Grant (Eds.), *Alcohol and pleasure: A health perspective* (pp. 11–23). Philadelphia: Brunner/Mazel.

Wiens, F., Zitzmann, A., Lachance M.-A., Yegles, M., Pragst, F., Wurst, F. M., et al. (2008). Chronic intake of fermented floral nectar by wild treeshrews. *Proceedings of the National Academy of Sciences of the United States of America, 105,* 10426–10431.

Willis, J. (2002). *Potent brews: A social history of alcohol in East Africa, 1850–1999.* Nairobi, Kenya: British Institute of East Africa.

Wilson, E. O. (2000). *Sociobiology: The new synthesis.* Cambridge, MA: Harvard University Press. (Original work published 1975)

Wiltermuth, S. S., & Heath, C. (2009). Synchrony and cooperation. *Psychological Science, 20,* 1–5.

Winslow, S., & Hall, S. (2006). *Violent night: Urban leisure and contemporary culture.* Oxford, UK: Berg.

Zahavi, A., & Zahavi, A. (1997). *The handicap principle: A missing piece of Darwin's puzzle.* Oxford, UK: Oxford University Press.

4

Drunkenness—A Historical and Contemporary Cross-Cultural Perspective: "A Voluntary Madness"

Fiona Measham

Accounts from many countries demonstrate how the experiences, behaviors, meanings, and significance of drunkenness and responses to degrees of drunkenness are firmly located in time and place. This chapter considers, from an interdisciplinary perspective, competing and contrasting understandings of drunkenness alongside an overview of historical and contemporary debates on its definitions and measurements. The central focus throughout this chapter, as in this book in general, is on the experiences and behaviors related to *acute* alcohol consumption, variously referred to as *drunkenness, intoxication, binge drinking, extreme drinking,* or *heavy episodic drinking,* and on how historically these terms have been defined and understood—rather than on chronic, daily, or dependent drinking. As we shall come to see, the reason why such behaviors are being studied is as salient a question as what is studied or how.

In this chapter, historical and cross-cultural overviews of recent perspectives on drunkenness and binge drinking, a term currently favored in many academic and policy circles, show both the proliferation and amorphousness of drunken behavior. A consideration of the contemporary debate on drunkenness and binge drinking explores the relationship among intoxication, beverage choice, drinking venues, and promotional practices, alongside drinkers' own perceptions of alcohol consumption, excess, and moderation across Europe and North America. A case study of the Australian phenomenon known as the *six o'clock swill* provides a glimpse of drunkenness in a cultural context that has sanctioned such behavior and draws attention to the extent such historically engrained drinking patterns can be changed through intervention. This Anglo-Saxon example is then compared to the experiences of several European countries, where attitudes and behaviors relating to heavy drinking appear to be converging, and to Japanese and Chinese societies, where historically public drunkenness has been rarely socially sanctioned, but where now there are emergent trends of both increased and reduced tolerance toward such behaviors among male drinking groups.

We begin with a consideration of historical perspectives on drunkenness to illustrate how cultural differences in attitudes are rooted in historical precedents with respect to excessive drinking and to the broader social, religious, spiritual, and political values within which such attitudes and behaviors can be contextualized.

THE HISTORICAL ROOTS OF THE CONTEMPORARY DRUNKENNESS DEBATE

One of the challenges of trying to define, understand, and assess the cultural significance of any concept is the sheer number of words in any given language to discuss it. As Heath (2000, p. 125) noted, in most languages, we find a scale of words denoting levels of drunkenness, from *tipsy* to *blotto,* or *dead drunk,* each level conveying different expectations of behavior and often different degrees of social approval or disapproval. Lay descriptions of drunkenness used in the past are equally evocative; *cut and fuddled, chuck-full, bosky, crooks his elbow,* and *got a crumb in his beard* are some of the 80 epithets for drunkenness listed by Thomas Norwood in the 1770 *Gentleman's Magazine,* demonstrating that bouts of heavy drinking have been common in England for centuries (quoted in Clark, 1983, pp. 277–278). Levine (1981) noted that the 1975 *Dictionary of American Slang* contained more synonyms for the word *drunk* (353 terms) than for any other entry, and the *American Thesaurus of Slang* included a staggering 900 terms for *drunk* (p. 1038). This "linguistic friction," as Midanik (2003, p. 1286) described it, is indicative of the pervasiveness of not only drinking, but also drunkenness to the human condition.

The meaning and significance of a particular term can evolve or be extended over time. In English, the term *binge drinking* can be traced to the mid-19th century, when it was included in *A Glossary of Northamptonshire Words and Phrases; with Examples of Their Colloquial Use:* "A man goes to the alehouse to get a good binge, or to binge himself" (Baker, 1854/2003, p. 49). The origins of the word *binge,* however, lie further back in the English dialect. According to the *Oxford English Dictionary,* it meant "to soak a wooden vessel." Applied to alcohol, this implied drinking to a point of feeling soaked, indicative of bloating and excess even in the word's earliest application. Today, the definition of binge remains contested, as discussed later.

The language of intoxication can reveal differences between cultures and tell us how people experience this altered state. In a study of language used to describe intoxication in five European cities, Cameron and colleagues (2000) found that English, Dutch, and Swedish respondents tended to define it in terms of negative behaviors; Greeks spoke of intoxication in psychological terms of "transformation"; and Scottish respondents evoked both psychological definitions and negative behavioral outcomes for the extreme levels of drunkenness. There are many such broad categorizations of nations and societies based on their relationship to alcohol.

In the past, as today, comparisons have been drawn between the drunkenness of populations in the northern climes and the more measured drinking patterns of southern Europeans, traditionally perceived as more rarely drinking to intoxication (or drunkenness). Barr (1995) argued that heavy drinking has always been part of the British character, distinguishing the inhabitants of the United Kingdom from their continental neighbors. He referred to the 8th-century missionary and reformer Saint Boniface, born in Britain but living most of his life in Europe; in his old age, Boniface wrote to Cuthbert, the Archbishop of Canterbury, "In your dioceses, the vice of drunkenness is too frequent. This is an evil peculiar to pagans and to our race. Neither the Franks nor the Gauls nor the Lombards nor the Romans nor the Greeks commit it" (quoted in Barr, 1995, p. 25). According to some accounts, drunkenness became a national characteristic or an attribute of particular cultural groups due to a long historical process.

In an examination of Soviet and American heavy-drinking cultures, Segal (1986) contended that patterns of excessive alcohol consumption in late 20th-century Russia and among Irish Americans had been preceded by, and were the outcome of, many sociocultural and psychobiological factors building up over the centuries and resulting in social dissonance, with individuals feeling growing alienation, anxiety, boredom, narcissism, and loss of a sense of belonging. Alexander (2004) went further by describing addiction as the predominant way of adapting to feelings of dislocation and lack of psychosocial integration found in all modern free-market consumer societies (see also James, 2007, 2008). Similar explanations have been proposed for young people's binge drinking—that it is a manifestation of social exclusion and boredom. There is a consensus, however, among both researchers and social commentators that, for British youth and young adults, drunkenness can be premeditated, functional (e.g., carnivalesque, as discussed later), and widespread rather than simply the hedonistic pursuit of a deviant, disadvantaged, or deprived minority (Measham & Brain, 2005; Parker, Aldridge, & Measham, 1998; Parker & Williams, 2003; Szmigin et al., 2008; see also Chapter 5).

The functionality of alcohol consumption is a persistent theme in past research, with drunkenness itself not always regarded as socially unacceptable. Porter (1985) reminded us that, in Europe, the dominant response to drunkenness before the 19th century was "generalised disapproval," and that it was prized as "manly" in Georgian England. Levine (1984) commented that most colonials in 18th-century America "regarded drunkenness as unproblematic and unsurprising; drunkenness was seen as the natural, normal and harmless result of drinking" (p. 110). Anthropological studies commonly describe drinking to intoxication as part of rituals and carnivals in many societies (see Chapter 3), a custom that survives to the present day in celebrations such as the Mardi Gras in Rio de Janeiro, Brazil. Similarly, drunkenness by young people can be seen as calculated theater that has occurred on the streets of countries such as the United Kingdom on Friday and Saturday nights for decades, if not centuries (A. Davies, 1992; Pearson, 1983; Presdee, 2000; Tuck, 1989), and, indeed, has become a subject for regular recycling on reality television programs (Hayward & Hobbs, 2007). As Borsay (2007; see also Presdee, 2000) suggested,

> We need to understand more the thrill and excitement of the occasion, the frisson generated by engaging in what is essentially carnivalesque behaviour in which the social norms are challenged and inverted. We need to look more at the performative aspects of binge-drinking. . . . Young people are performing before a virtual audience. However, they do so fully in the knowledge that it is only carnival, that during the week they will return to their normal lives. In this sense binge-drinking, as in pre-modern

> Carnival, simply reaffirms the norms of society by temporarily challenging them. (p. 3)

There are various explanations for why drunkenness is tolerated and even encouraged in some circumstances. Intoxication is a required state in some religious rituals where communication with the gods can only be achieved through altered consciousness induced by the use of alcohol or drugs (Heath, 2000, p. 126). Horton (1943), studying the functions of alcohol in "primitive" societies, suggested that alcohol offered a way of coping with tension, unhappiness, and frustration, an anxiety-reducing function akin to a "time out" from the normal rigors and constraints of everyday life, described also by MacAndrew and Edgerton (1969/2003) in their work on drunken comportment in early societies. Discussing precolonial Latin America, Rosovsky (1999) stated that, "Some societies, such as the Mapuche, included deliberate and socially accepted drunkenness as part of celebrations related to economic transactions, marriages, or the meting out of justice" (p. 90). Similarly, Clark (1983) noted the role of alcohol in formalizing both business and nuptial arrangements in medieval and early modern Britain. Drinking to intoxication has also been observed to signify positions of power and status. In early Mexican society, it helped to define collective identity; in modern Mestizo culture, feats of competitive drinking accompanied by insults and fighting continued as a form of self-assertion (Douglas, 1987). Again, we have only to think of student drinking games—such as American fraternity and sorority rites of passage (Kilmer & Larimer, 2008; Wechsler, Kuh, & Davenport, 1996)—to see the survival and symbolic value of competitive drinking and drunkenness.

Examples from anthropological and cross-cultural studies clearly indicate, then, that drinking with the intention of becoming drunk is not a new phenomenon, and, contrary to dominant media images of our times, it is not confined to the young. However, as discussed in Chapter 1, a key component of drunkenness is the behavior associated with alcohol consumption—a result of subjective interpretations of expected or desired reactions to alcohol as well as the actual physiological state of intoxication, bounded by social and cultural constraints that define what is or is not acceptable in a particular society or social group. Put simply, people learn how to drink and how to behave when drunk. As classic anthropological studies have shown (e.g., MacAndrew & Edgerton, 1969/2003), drunken comportment takes many forms, from aggression and violence—even in normally peaceful peoples—to gaiety and euphoria or passivity and sleep. With respect to concerns about heavy episodic drinking and the outcomes of acute consumption-related attitudes and behaviors (see, e.g., Martinic & Measham, 2008), researchers in a growing number of countries around the world have identified a pattern of intentional drunkenness or *extreme drinking* among certain groups of young people. This often takes place outside traditionally defined and approved social occasions and involves ways of behaving defined by the young themselves as appropriate but seen by wider social groups—public health professionals, parents, politicians, and the media—as inappropriate. What remains unchanged in many of these countries is the concern expressed by the authorities about the high visibility, to both critics and participants, of public drunkenness and the age and gender of drinkers (Jayne, Valentine, & Holloway, 2008; Measham & Østergaard, 2009).

Even in societies where alcohol is allowed and drunkenness is condoned or tolerated, boundaries are placed on who can drink, how much, and when. Permission to become drunk (at whatever level) is not granted to everyone. Acceptance of drunkenness often signifies attaining a desired status, such as coming of age—or, in modern times, reaching the age when the purchase of alcohol becomes legal. In many societies, permission to get drunk has been reserved for those in a position of authority or privilege. For example, Brennan (1991) described how increasing access to wine underpinned elite condemnation of drunkenness in Old Regime Paris: "This official literature [on drunkenness] . . . reveals the secret of a rage among the upper classes at seeing a social distinction diminish in a consumption from which they hoped the poor would remain excluded as a sign of inferior condition" (p. 69).

Women and Drunkenness

In many societies, slaves, serfs, young people, and women have been commonly refused alcohol or restricted in their consumption. Among the Lele in Zaire, for instance, there is social disapproval of drunkenness because it indicates a lack of self-control and sharing. However, a distinction is made between degrees of drunkenness, with tipsiness being accepted in men but not women; becoming tipsy is associated with masculine attributes such as aggressiveness and assertiveness, leading to the suppression of inhibitions—regarded as inappropriate for women (Ngokwey, 1987).

We can use women's alcohol consumption to illustrate some of the many factors shaping drunkenness. In all societies, women have used mood-altering substances, but we rarely find cultures in which they are culturally permitted to participate in substance use on equal terms with men, and there are restrictions on female drinking in most cultures (Gefou-Madianou, 1992; Roche et al., 2007). One exception comes in ancient Egypt, where "Women, particularly of the upper class, appeared to have had unlimited access to alcohol as society's acceptance of alcoholic beverages increased. Banquet scriptures encouraged them to join in and 'not spoil the entertainment'" (El-Guebaly & El-Guebaly, 1981, p. 1207). In other societies, women were banned from drinking altogether. There may be little truth in the story that a Roman woman had to greet her male relatives with a kiss to prove she had not been drinking, but Jellinek (1976) recorded the existence of a law in early Rome forbidding women to drink, most probably, he speculated, to safeguard patrimonial rights (see also Chapter 3). More commonly, women have faced heavier constraints and sanctions on alcohol consumption than men, and intoxication in women, especially maternal drunkenness, has almost always attracted social disapproval (Foster, 1995; Plant, 1997; Stockley, 1998). Ettorre (1997) documented the multiple negative images attached to drunken women—"the drunken whore, the loose woman, the female lush, the weak woman, the evil woman, . . . the bad mother, the out-of-control woman"—commenting that such images pigeonholed female drinkers into a single category of "disgraceful woman" (p. 91).

The stigmatization of drunkenness in women can be traced through the centuries and across cultures. In England, for instance, from Hogarth's famous depiction of the drunken mother during the 18th-century gin craze (Measham, 2008), we move to 19th-century fears of maternal drinking (and drug use) as a cause of infant deaths and national degeneration (Berridge, 1981), to early 20th-century worries about "modern girls" with financial and social independence and a tendency to a hedonistic lifestyle that included immoderate alcohol (and drug) use (Kohn, 1992, 1997), and finally to the "ladette" culture of today, typified by binge drinking, badly behaved young women (Jackson & Tinkler, 2007). It has been argued that intoxication in women, often linked to sexual freedom or abandonment and the neglect of children and household responsibilities, arouses social anxieties and condemnation because it represents a threat to the traditional social order and a threat to the health and well-being of children and, therefore, of the nation as a whole. As McDonald (1994) noted in her account of alcohol consumption in traditional Breton culture, it is often a woman's job to control male drinking (as well as her own); thus, intoxication by women represents a relinquishing of the role of "moral architects and guardians of social order" (p. 112). It was not until the Middle Ages, however, that temperance as a specifically feminine virtue emerged, concurrent with growing tensions over scarce resources in postplague and famine Europe.

Gender is, of course, only one of the factors that determined the boundaries of drunkenness across centuries. In relation to drunkenness, the point here is that both formal and informal controls, including regulation at national and local levels, have tended to strengthen over time and varied from place to place. When legislation and controls on drunkenness have been introduced, it is often because of concerns over public disorder, fears of political instability, and the perceived relationship among drinking venues, drunkenness, and threats to authority. According to some historical accounts, as the alehouses of 16th-century England were increasingly frequented by the lower classes, they became the focus of a concerted offensive linked to the rise of Protestantism, the fear of political instability, and a determination to control the threat of an uprising (Clark, 1983). Conversely, the rise of Protestantism was also linked to the development of temperance movements across Europe and North America (Gusfield, 1986; Harrison, 1971). A similar analysis of reactions to drunkenness in France in the same period was discussed by Brennan (1991), although, as the author pointed out, the laws and punishments were only fitfully carried out. Where punishments were declared, they were often severe. In 16th-century France, imprisonment on a diet of bread and water was meted out for a first offense, followed by whipping for subsequent offenses (Brennan, 1991). In England, being sent to the stocks, fines, and whipping were seen as appropriate responses to public drunkenness (Williams & Brake, 1980). In many countries, sermons against drunkenness helped to establish the moral boundaries around drinking and to define excess consumption as a sin leading to idleness, blasphemy, homicides, and other social ills—although the relationship between cause and effect was often unclear (see, e.g., Brennan, 1991, p. 68). Indeed, disapproval of excessive drinking in Europe and North America came primarily from the clergy, whose members associated it with the sin of gluttony (Bennett, 1991, p. 176; Warner, 1997, p. 99).

We can see, then, how contemporary attitudes toward drunkenness and excess have been shaped by the historical and cultural contexts. The experience, meaning, and significance of drunkenness, its outcomes, and social responses are also products of cultural evolution.

THE CONTEMPORARY DRUNKENNESS DEBATE

Historically, in discussions of drinking, a distinction has been made between, first, excessive consumption during a drinking session that results in drunkenness and associated risks to the individual, the community, and wider society, and, second, heavy drinking across a much longer period that leads to alcohol dependence or alcoholism (and a different set of associated risks). Furthermore, drunkenness has had an added distinction from alcoholism in its greater emphasis on choice, personal responsibility, or agency that facilitates the potential for individual self-control, as distinct from the "disease" of alcoholism with its implied helplessness and conceptualization in Western medicine as a problem in need of medical assessment and intervention (J. B. Davies, 1997). This emphasis on individual choice, moral responsibility, and, therefore, individual resolution in relation to drunkenness was emphasized as long ago as the early 18th century in an anonymous 1705 English pamphlet that described drunkenness as "a Sin which hath long been called a Voluntary Madness" (quoted in Babor, 1994, p. 1128).* From the late 18th century onward, the notion that drunkenness was the leading cause of insanity gradually gained hold across the Western world, a belief eagerly popularized by temperance reformers but instigated and perpetuated by the medical profession from the early 19th century at a time of limited understanding of mental illness and psychiatric disorders (McCandless, 1984). Indeed, in McCandless's (1984) account of the close relationship between the medical profession and temperance reformers, he suggested that "medical men provided the Temperance Movement with many of its most powerful weapons against alcohol" (p. 51). Temperance advocates eagerly and without question repeated

* It was not until the late 18th century, however, that the "discovery of addiction" as a disease or medical condition relating to chronic, dependent drinking started to develop (Levine, 1978).

inaccurate statistics on drunkenness as the main cause of insanity. Historically, such concerns had an economic context: Differential taxation meant spirits were proportionately cheaper and more potent than traditional wines and ales, leading to concerns about increased drinking, increased drunkenness, and increased alcohol-related health, social, and public order problems (McCandless, 1984; see also Warner, 2003).

The historical concerns about the relationship between drunkenness and changing beverage preferences and, in particular, the emergence of "new" higher potency drinks have their echoes in the recent *alcopops* debate.* Flavored alcohol beverages and ready-to-drink spirit mixers were popularized in the European alcohol market from the 1990s onward (Brain & Parker, 1997; Forsyth, 2001). Concerns were expressed that the combined potency and sweetness of the new drinks might make them appealing to youthful and female tastes. Although the high price of the so-called alcopops in the 1990s meant that the first wave of drinkers were as likely to be those over 18 as those under that age, the consumption of alcopops has increased among young people in recent years. For example, there was a rise in the reported consumption of alcopops on last drinking occasion among secondary school students between a survey conducted in 1999 and a follow-up survey 4 years later in the United Kingdom, Belgium, Cyprus, Denmark, Greece, Greenland, Ireland, the Isle of Man, the Netherlands, and Norway, with an average of 12% of last-occasion alcohol consumption accounted for by alcopops (Hibell et al., 2004, p. 343).† In the United Kingdom, for example, this figure increased from 16% (in 1999) to 31% (in 2003) of

* The term *alcopops* was originally applied as shorthand for alcoholic lemonades or "pops"—such as *Two Dogs,* developed in Australia in the early 1990s and launched in Europe in the mid-1990s—it is now used by alcohol researchers (e.g., Hibell et al., 2004) and nonstatutory and public-sector organizations (e.g., Alcohol Concern, 2001; Goddard, 2007) to denote a wide range of flavored alcoholic beverages (FABs), ready-to-drink spirit or malt-based drinks (RTDs), and other new alcohol drinks that have developed since then. Some alcohol advocacy organizations, politicians, and the media have portrayed these products as purposefully designed to tempt underage young people (Brain & Parker, 1997; Forsyth, 2001). Not surprisingly, manufacturers and retailers prefer the terms *FABs* or *RTDs* to *alcopops.*

† The European School Survey Project on Alcohol and Other Drugs (ESPAD) conducts ongoing surveys in secondary schools across Europe at 4-year intervals. Four data collections have been published to date (1995, 1999, 2003, and 2007). The first study was conducted in 26 countries in 1995 and was later expanded to more than 100,000 high school students in 35 countries. These surveys provide detailed comparative analyses of drinking, as well as smoking and drug use, among 15- to 16-year-olds, using randomly selected classes from a nationally representative sample.

15-year-old girls and from 9% to 17% of 15-year-old boys (Hibell et al., 2004).

The suggested relationship between beverage choice and the subsequent amount consumed—with more potent drinks leading to higher levels of intoxication—is nothing new, of course. It was the central point in Hogarth's classic 18th-century engravings that compared the rosy consequences of beer drinking in *Beer Street* with the pitiful consequences of gin drinking, depicted as the downfall of men, women, and children in *Gin Lane,* in what could be considered the first popular national alcohol health promotion campaign nearly 300 years ago. More recently, however, research has suggested that several factors have facilitated a growing tendency among significant numbers of young people to heavy episodic drinking and drinking to drunkenness, including the following:

- The higher potency of drinks available.
- More frequent mixing of drinks.
- The growing popularity of shots, shooters, or "chasers."
- Increased "preloading" with cheap drinks bought in shops and consumed at home before a night out (Hughes, Anderson, Morleo, & Bellis, 2007; Martinic & Measham, 2008; McKeganey, 1998; McKeganey, Forsyth, Barnard, & Hay, 1996; Measham & Brain, 2005).

Not only is drunkenness linked to the types of beverage alcohol preferred by certain individuals and their patterns of consumption, but quantity of alcohol consumed also appears to be associated with both specific licensed premises and the retail practices within them. Stockwell and colleagues (1992) found that higher numbers of drunken customers left from "high-risk" bars (defined by the ratio of measurable harm to alcohol sales in an individual bar) than from "low-risk" bars. This led the authors to conclude that "an effective approach to reducing alcohol-related accidents and injuries might be to reduce the incidence of high levels of intoxication on licensed premises" through the identification and targeting of interventions in "high-risk" licensed premises (Stockwell et al., 1992, p. 880). By focusing on specific premises, Stockwell et al. argued, it is possible to reach those customers who are more likely to drink to higher levels of intoxication—in other words, there is a strong relationship between premises and intoxication levels. Furthermore, a study of American college student drinking by Thombs and colleagues (2008) found that bar customers who reported having taken advantage of promotional offers were more than four times more likely to leave licensed premises with a blood alcohol concentration (BAC) above the American legal limit to drive* than customers who did not take advantage of the special offers in the same establishments. Of further note is that there was no significant gender difference in the BAC levels of this student sample.

Some definitions of drunkenness suggest that there is a sliding scale of stages or degrees of drunkenness. In other definitions, drunkenness is a clearly demarcated state that a drinker either does or does not achieve, exemplified in the quote attributed to the American "Rat Pack" actor and socialite Dean Martin: "You're not drunk if you can lie on the floor without holding on." Qualitative research exploring definitions of drunkenness suggests that, although there is an association between drinkers' perceptions of drunkenness and the number of drinks they consume, this definition varies from individual to individual, with gender, ethnicity, and social and cultural expectations also playing a part (see also Chapter 5). A study by Midanik (2003) used quantitative data for 1,366 current drinkers and qualitative data from a separate sample of 58 current drinkers to explore definitions and measurements of drunkenness. The quantitative data looked at the relationship between two indicators—frequency of drunkenness and number of drinks to feel drunk—whereas the qualitative data looked at drinkers' own definitions of drunkenness. Respondents identified six key criteria for being drunk:

- 26% of participants mentioned physiological symptoms (e.g., headaches, nausea).
- 26% referred to mobility (e.g., being unsafe to drive or feeling unsteady when walking).
- 16% talked about control issues (e.g., negative disinhibition, feeling "out of control").
- 15% listed positive outcomes (e.g., positive disinhibition, relaxation, taking a "time out" from everyday life).
- 9% emphasized speech symptoms (e.g., slurring words, verbal disinhibition).

* With a measured BAC level of over 0.8 mg/ml.

- 8% referred to cognition (e.g., impaired thought processes, vulnerability).

It is perhaps surprising to note that only 15% of the qualitative sample mentioned positive outcomes. However, when looking at the relationship between the respondents' self-reported frequency of drunkenness and their key criteria for drunkenness, positive definitions were more likely to come from individuals who themselves got drunk more frequently, whereas the more negative criteria such as loss of control were more likely to come from those who reported rarely getting drunk. Although it may not be surprising that people who enjoy an activity may participate in it more frequently, or that their self-definition of that activity is more likely to include positive criteria, the association between definitions of drunkenness and individual consumption levels does clearly demonstrate the socially and culturally embedded nature of both the experience and the concept of contemporary drunkenness.

In what could be considered a companion to Midanik's study, Green, Polen, Janoff, Castleton, and Perrin (2007) explored perceptions of moderate drinking. For some respondents, moderation was, by definition, when the drinker did not feel drunk, regardless of the volume consumed and one's tolerance or predilection for alcohol, and therefore *moderate drinking* was a flexible concept for some respondents that potentially could involve increasing amounts of alcohol as individual tolerance increased. For others, moderation was the absence of the short-term negative consequences usually associated with episodes of heavy drinking, or the lack of dependency problems—again regardless of the actual amount consumed. The question posed by the work of Midanik, Green, and colleagues is how to frame alcohol education, information, and interventions when subjective perceptions of drunkenness, sobriety, or cognitive and behavioral functioning may be above or below "official" moderate-drinking recommendations, and might not necessarily relate to either a clear linear relationship or correlation with units of alcohol consumed. Yet, in many countries, the working definitions of moderate and immoderate drinking are simple unit-based thresholds set as a result of medical research on the increased risk of health problems above certain levels of alcohol intake.

What is clear (and of concern to Green et al., 2007) is how individualized such definitions of moderation are and how they incorporate the recognition of the influence of gender, body mass index, and other factors. There is thus a disdain among some drinkers for what might be deemed simplistic population-based public health messages about sensible consumption. On the positive side, it could be that the general public can understand and, indeed, prefers more accurate and more sophisticated public health messages that can be applied to drinkers' own circumstances. In the field of illicit drugs, by contrast, the subjectivities of the experience of intoxication are well recognized, as, for example, in the classic text on "drug, set, and setting" (Zinberg, 1984), which outlined how a drug's effects are determined not solely by the drug dose itself, nor even the dosage interacting with the individual user's physiology, but also by the "mind-set" of the user and the wider sociocultural "setting" or environment for use. This phenomenon has also been demonstrated in animal experiments: Alexander (1985), in a series of tests that came to be known as the *Rat Park experiments,* demonstrated how less stressful and more stimulating environments decreased patterns of self-administered substance use in rats (see also Chapter 3). Similarly with alcohol then, we would expect the composite experience of drunkenness to relate to far more than simply the number of drink units consumed, but also to factors relating to the individual drinker, his or her mind-set, the localized drinking environment or community, and the broader sociocultural setting. To distinguish moderate from excessive consumption and bring clarity to the complex, subjective, and culturally embedded notions of drunkenness already discussed, use of the term *binge drinking* has emerged in recent debates.

THE CONTEMPORARY BINGE DRINKING DEBATE

As previously noted, the meaning and use of the term *binge* has shifted in recent times. So what is binge drinking, why does it exist, and why has it been so necessary to define it? A number of reviews (e.g., Herring, Berridge, & Thom, 2008; Plant & Plant, 2006) have highlighted the shifts in use of the term from colloquialisms such as "being soaked in alcohol" to clinical definitions that involved drinking to intoxication over a number of days (the popular notion of "going on a bender"), and through to more recent definitions focused on a single drinking session with a specified number of units of alcohol consumed* (Wechsler, Davenport, Dowdall, Moeykens, & Castillo, 1994; Wechsler, Dowdall, Davenport, & Castillo, 1995; Wechsler et al., 1996) or on frequency of self-perceived drunkenness (Midanik, 1999; Richardson & Budd, 2003). Yet, these recent attempts to quantify moderate and immoderate levels of drinking have failed to distinguish between the behaviors and risks of the different sociodemographic groups the term has been applied to—for example, young women (Jackson & Tinkler, 2007) and underage youth (Coleman & Cater, 2003, 2005; Squires, 2008). It is also important to note that uses of the term *binge* have been displaced rather than replaced in these various clinical, popular, political, and policy-oriented contexts, and remain contested.

The clinical definition of a binge encompassed an extended period of time (typically at least 2 days) in which a person repeatedly becomes intoxicated and gives up his or her usual activities and obligations to do so (Schuckit, 1998). As noted earlier, the threshold for unit-based binge drinking was set in response to health concerns and therefore included the drinking behavior of a significant minority of the young adult population. Establishing a single threshold of a given number of units (differentiated only by gender) was open to criticism for failing to recognize the complexities in drinking-related and drunkenness-related behaviors and risks. Although the unit-based definition has been increasingly favored in academic and policy discussions in the early 21st century, Midanik (2003) argued that such "researcher-driven" unit-based measures have proved less useful than the "respondent-driven" self-perceived drunkenness measures in identifying alcohol-related harm because drinkers "are the best judges of what level of alcohol can cause impairment" (p. 1287; see also Midanik, 1999). For example, in the United Kingdom at the height of public concerns about young adult binge drinking, the official "moderate" drinking threshold was so broad as to result in nearly half of young men and over a

* In the United States, a binge has been officially defined as having five or more drinks for men and four or more drinks for women on a given occasion (Wechsler & Isaac, 1992; Wechsler, Davenport, Dowdall, Moeykens, & Castillo, 1994). In the United Kingdom, a binge is usually defined as drinking double the recommended daily sensible drinking maximum in a single drinking session. In terms of quantity of alcohol consumed, in the United States, a standard drink unit contains 14 g of pure alcohol, so a "bingeing" man would need to consume five drinks (equivalent to 70 g of alcohol) at a sitting, and a "bingeing" woman would need to consume four drinks (56 g). By comparison, in the United Kingdom, a unit contains 8 g of pure alcohol, so binge drinking is defined as having 64 g of alcohol (eight units) for a man and 48 g of alcohol (six units) for a woman.

third of young women in 2004 (48% of men and 39% of women 16–24 years old) drinking above daily recommendations of four or three units, respectively, in the previous week (Goddard & Green, 2005). This led to concerns that a "credibility gulf" might develop between widespread drinking practices and public health messages, particularly if the pleasure of drunkenness itself was the goal (Measham, 2006). However, frequency of feeling the effects of alcohol is a poor predictor of health and social problems, or dependency (Midanik, 1999), as potentially one drinker could binge drink (by the unit-based definition) across a protracted drinking session and still feel relatively sober (Martinic & Measham, 2008), whereas another could drink within sensible guidelines and feel drunk (Midanik, 2003). Midanik concluded that, rather than the net already being cast too wide with detrimental effects in terms of credibility (Measham, 2006), it should be cast even wider to reduce the likelihood of missing some at-risk individuals who drink to drunkenness but within the sensible drinking recommendations (Wechsler et al., 1995), arguing that the focus of public health should be drunkenness rather than intoxication.

Most recently, and in recognition of the limitations and confusions surrounding the various clinical, unit-based, and user-based definitions of binge, there has been a policy shift away from these unit-based definitions. So, for example, in an overview of the British alcohol strategy, binge drinking was defined as "essentially drinking too much alcohol over a short period of time, e.g., over the course of an evening, and it is typically *drinking that leads to drunkenness*" (Department of Health, Home Office, Department for Education and Skills, & Department for Culture, Media and Sport, 2007, p. 3, italics added). In this definition, drunkenness is presented as the outcome of binge drinking, and, therefore, Midanik's at-risk individuals drinking within recommended limits could also be classified as binge drinkers. This shift from quantitative measures to subjective outcomes of drunkenness could potentially result in a lowering of the number of units specified in sensible-drinking recommendations, resulting in a widening of the net in terms of who is included in definitions of excessive consumption. Moreover, this shift from the objective to the subjective potentially results in the problematizing of drunkenness per se, as opposed to the problematizing of the risky outcomes of drinking above a certain level. Therefore, expanding the definition of binge drinking inflates the extent of the social problem and does not bring clarity to the debate, serving to confuse the general public and to increase the "credibility gulf" between drinkers and public health recommendations.

Like Midanik, Knupfer (1984) has questioned the merits of unit-based measures of drunkenness, arguing that the quantity of alcohol consumed per drinking session is far less significant than the frequency of intoxication (e.g., per week or month). At heart, she saw the focus on amount of alcohol consumed reflecting an "unwillingness to deal with the concept of drunkenness" (Knupfer, 1984, p. 186). In her analysis of the relationship between the prevalence of drinking problems and different indicators of frequency of drunkenness in nine population samples, she found that values, customs, and the tolerance or social acceptability of drunkenness varied, even within one society (the United States). Age, income, and marital status were not found to influence the acceptability of drunkenness; the only association in Knupfer's research was between gender and drunkenness (Knupfer, 1984, p. 195). In another study, Leigh (1984) identified age as a key variable, finding that among young people under 25 years old, drunkenness was not considered irresponsible or shameful, and any minor negative outcomes were approached with amusement rather than concern.

The binge drinking debate in contemporary Western societies is indicative of changing patterns of consumption, within the context of shifting cultural factors, such as:

- *Work:* Longer working hours leading to greater stress.
- *Leisure:* A "weekday restraint/weekend excess" Protestant work ethic evident in industrial and postindustrial countries since the late 18th century (Measham, 2008; this has been compounded since the 1950s by a growing emphasis, especially among young people, on the performance and maintenance of identity within a shortened leisure time that has led to a "living for the weekend" binge mentality—see Demant & Østergaard, 2007; Jarvinen & Room, 2007).
- *Delay in traditional life stages:* This includes prolonged economic dependence on parents, extended engagement in higher education, and later onset of parenthood (for review, see Roche et al., 2007).

Across a range of cultural groups in both developed and developing countries, there is evidence to suggest that some young people in recent years have embarked on an increasingly purposeful pursuit of the pleasures of drunkenness, choosing to get drunk in social situations as part of a broader, heightened emphasis on hedonistic consumption-oriented leisure and the pursuit of a "controlled loss of control" (Measham, 2002). This is seen in, for example, the recent emergence and rapid expansion of the *botellón** in public squares across Spain (see Bascones Perez-Fragero, 2008, pp. 193–197) and the well-established excessive consumption patterns of American sorority and fraternity students (Kilmer & Larimer, 2008, pp. 228–232). The comparative research suggests that this *extreme drinking* (a term introduced by Martinic & Measham, 2008) is both "calculated" in terms of individual motivation to achieve drunkenness (see also Featherstone, 1991; Szmigin et al., 2008) and "bounded" by the sociodemographic, cultural, and economic contexts of such consumption (see also Measham & Brain, 2005). Although this drinking pattern is more recent in some non-beer-drinking countries without a Protestant temperance tradition, in others, the historical roots of publicly condoned drunkenness are far more embedded in the cultural practices of particular social groups, as the Australian situation in Case Study 4.1 illustrates.

CASE STUDY 4.1: A Peculiarly Australian Phenomenon: The Six O'Clock Swill

Billie Atanasova

> "When I arrived in 1981 'shouts' were still very much the name of the game and the culture of the six o'clock swill remained."
>
> **Chuck Hahn,**
> *Chief Brewer of the Australian-American Lion Nathan Group*

A DRUNKEN CULTURE?

Alcohol consumption is embedded in Australian society and entrenched in much of its social life. It is used to mark key events such as births, deaths, marriage, graduation, promotions, and loss of a job (e.g., Roche et al., 2007). Traditionally, displays of intoxication have

* A phenomenon in Spain and, recently, some other countries (e.g., Switzerland) that involves large gatherings of mostly young people meeting outdoors to drink and socialize.

been tolerated, accepted, and even expected as a norm in many social contexts, whether these norms involve falling into a state of complete unconsciousness at a backyard barbecue or slightly losing one's balance while walking through a black-tie gala event. Australians have a reputation for heavy drinking, a reputation that has deep historical roots. To understand how this national image was first established, it is necessary to refer to the sociocultural history of alcohol in Australia and, in particular, a peculiarly Australian phenomenon known as the *six o'clock swill.*

Anglo-Celtic Baggage?

A reputation for heavy drinking has been part of White Australia's national image from the Rum Corps* at the beginning of British colonization to drunkenness among gold diggers, to the lasting traditions of bush workers' "shouts" and the end-of-week "work and burst" drunken blowouts (Room, 1988). In the early colonial history, spirits were used as currency, and convicts were paid partially in rum (Lewis, 1992). The role of alcohol in the country's history has been noted by many writers—for example, as Lewis (1997/2006) observed, "Heavy drinking has had a central place in Australian social life from the time of the First Fleet"† (p. 1).

Associated with this image of heavy drinking has been "the ideology of male 'mateship,' the strong commitment to mutual support and cohesion and egalitarian relations in groups drawn or thrown together in work parties, in sports or other play" (Room, 1988, p. 414). The predominantly male preserve of heavy drinking in Australian history was central to various rituals of male solidarity (Lewis, 1992); women, non-European immigrants, and indigenous people were excluded from this "mateship" nationalistic drinking culture (Kirkby, 2003). So, contrary to the popular stereotype, Horne (1964) acknowledged that Australians have never been quite the nation of boozers they imagine themselves

* The military force stationed in New South Wales (NSW) from 1792 to 1810, the NSW Corps, was nicknamed the Rum Corps because of its monopoly on the spirits trade. The Corps played a key role in the Rum Rebellion of 1808, the only successful military coup in Australia's recorded history.

† The First Fleet refers to 11 ships that sailed from Great Britain in 1787 to establish the first European colony, a convict settlement, in New South Wales.

to be, and that, in a significant proportion of the population, the myths remained just that.

The traditional focus of Australian drinking was the hotel or the pub. Getting drunk was what many Australians equated with the "the good life." There was a degree of tolerance for scenes such as that described by Kirkby (2003):

> The streets filled with wild cries and the gutters ran with chunder … legless drunks … staggering up the street, barking at the pavement, cannoning off the buildings and plate glass, crawling on their hands and knees that last few yards to their cars. (p. 246)

Following World War II, alcohol consumption rates increased substantially, peaking in the 1970s but steadily declining thereafter. This change in drinking patterns is often attributed to the easing of controls on alcohol availability, combined with growing wine consumption from the late 1960s and the "general trends of cosmopolitanisation and the commodification and the privatization of leisure" (Room, 1988, p. 416; see also Roche et al., 2007). Many social historians have suggested that the easing of controls on alcohol availability contributed to the elimination of the "beer-guzzling frenzy and lively street scenes," or the six o'clock swill.*

The Six O'Clock Swill

The six o'clock swill is one of the best-known terms in Australian history. Its popularity encapsulates the pub drinking practices of a 50-year period from the Great War until the 1960s, when pubs closed at six o'clock in most Australian states.† The short period between the end of the working day and the pub's closing was called the six o'clock swill, when patrons would rush to "guzzle" as much beer as they could before the end of the day's serving (for an account of similar practices in the United Kingdom, see Tuck, 1989). The atmosphere and action were aptly conveyed by Dunstan (1968) in the novel *Wowsers:*

> [The pub is] a large room, with a cold lavatory-like atmosphere, but filled with pushing men. There are no seats, no tables, no stools, no clutter that might interfere with the high-speed action. … There are special

* The phenomenon has also been noted in New Zealand's historical drinking culture.

† Tasmania had a 10 p.m. closing time in 1937 and staggered hours during World War II, thus avoiding this phenomenon (Luckins, 2007).

> men and ladies on for the peak panic, eight or even ten immensely skilled barmen and barmaids, all equipped with the latest pluto taps on plastic hoses, an invention designed for dispensing beer at frightening speed, but they cannot cope. It is ten to six, now five to six, the bar is ten deep with pushing bodies, all thrusting handfuls of glasses towards the barmaids: "Here"—"Here"—"For Chrissake here." Well, you know this barmaid pretty well, she serves you first, but then you have to get your five glasses back to your mates against the wall … under the no-ornament-no-seat-no-comfort-all-action policy there were no tables, and while there were often ledges or windowsills, one had to get in early to make use of them. So the only choice was for each member of the school to put his five beers between his feet on the ground, and then demolish one by one before six. … But now it is two minutes to six, the mob is getting desperate, like the last few fighting for the lifeboats on a sinking ship. … At six the publican would ring bells, make announcements over an amplifier, he would go round almost with tears in his eyes urging everyone to finish their drinks: "Come on, fellers, fair go, drink up, fair go." … At 6:15 pm the crowd, after their 30 minutes or so of tension, would be out on the footpath, many reeling. Constitutions that have not known food for five hours or more need to be strong to take five beers in 30 minutes on an empty stomach. (pp. 100–101)

Although the six o'clock swill no longer exists in contemporary Australia, elements within the public health sector and the media might argue that remnants of this drinking practice still remain. The association of temperance with "wowserism"* has been an effective deterrent until recently when saying anything negative about alcohol and its availability. "The language is urgent, the message alarming: Alcohol is out of control, a silent time bomb, a silent epidemic" were the words used in a 2008 article in one of Australia's most respected newspapers ("Hitting the Drink," 2008, p. 15). The "binge drinking epidemic" and "public drunkenness out of control" are two of a flurry of slogans that have appeared in the Australian media, as with the British media, and have led to Australia's cultural predisposition to drunkenness becoming a governmental priority.

---

* Originally, this slang expression, used in Australia and New Zealand, meant "a lout"; this meaning shifted in the 1900s to denote a person who prevents others from their "sinful" pleasures, including drinking. The term was particularly applied to members of the temperance movement.

Case Study 4.1 raises important questions about the extent to which Australia's (or, indeed, any country's) drinking culture can be changed. The work of social historians allows an understanding of the embedded meanings of alcohol in Australian society, how the development and perpetuation of the six o'clock swill has shaped the boundaries of drunkenness and acceptability in modern Australia, and how the historical continuities of drinking to get drunk might be considered a form of national cultural expression, much in the same way as are the historical continuities of the British tradition of weekend drunkenness and weekday restraint (Clark, 1983; Gollancz, 1943/1972; Harrison, 1971; Measham, 2006; Measham & Brain, 2005). More recently, changing drinking patterns in Australia, as in other Anglo-Saxon countries, have enhanced these long-standing traditions: So, for example, the location and duration of the "drinking to get drunk" time frame has increased (from 5:30 or 6 p.m. to, say, 5:30 p.m. to 2 a.m. on a Friday or Saturday night), in conjunction with a sociodemographic broadening of gender, age, and ethnicity of drinkers and the expansion of the nighttime economy seen in many countries (Hadfield, 2009). Thus, recent changes in drinking-related attitudes and behaviors enhance long-standing Anglo-Saxon drinking traditions, combined with changing trends in migration and an increasingly culturally diverse population (Room, 2005).

CONVERGING PATTERNS OF DRINKING, DRUNKENNESS, AND ABSTENTION?

There is evidence of both a diversification and a convergence of drinking and drunkenness-related patterns and behaviors. In terms of convergence, the influence of "'ambivalent,' northern, beer-drinking cultures on 'integrated,' southern, wine-drinking cultures is increasing" (Social Issues Research Centre [SIRC], 1998, p. 11) and has led to growing concerns about alcohol-related health, social, and public safety problems associated with excessive drinking, particularly by young people (as noted in a review of the social and cultural aspects of drinking by SIRC, 1998). The European School Survey Project on Alcohol and Other Drugs (ESPAD) of 15- to 16-year-old students also supported this notion of convergence in experiences of drunkenness, at least among young people. The four ESPAD surveys to date suggest that, in general, frequent drinking, heavy drinking, and drunkenness are more common among teenage girls and boys in northern European countries such as Denmark, Finland, Ireland, the Netherlands, and the United Kingdom than in southern European countries such as France, Greece, Italy, and Portugal in terms of both subjective self-assessed drunkenness measures (e.g., self-reported lifetime, past-year, and past-month drunkenness) and unit-based heavy episodic drinking measures (e.g., Hibell et al., 2004). However, although alcohol consumption and drunkenness rates remain high among northern European teenagers, there is evidence of stability and decline in the most recently published ESPAD survey (Hibell et al., 2009). By contrast, in southern European countries that traditionally did not show such patterns of teenage consumption, a slight increase in frequent drinking, heavy drinking, and drunkenness has been reported. It has been noted that, although increased sessional consumption of beer in previously wine-drinking cultures in southern Europe (with traditionally lower levels of alcohol-related health and social problems) may lead to increased alcohol-related harm, a rise in wine consumption in previously beer-drinking cultures of northern Europe (with traditionally higher levels of alcohol-related health and social problems) has not led to a reduction in the incidence of harm (Measham & Østergaard, 2009), nor has it resulted in "the more harmonious behaviour and attitudes associated with wine-drinking cultures" (SIRC, 1998, p. 11). This suggests that the protective factors within a specific drinking culture are not necessarily easily replicated in a different cultural context.

Due to ambiguities and inconsistencies of the terminology and related public debate surrounding binge drinking, policymakers have been shifting their focus away from sessional consumption in public space by underage, young adult, and female drinkers toward a new concern for weekly consumption levels and home-based drinking, which incorporates older drinkers and professional occupational groups into the debate. Definitions of moderate and binge drinking focus more on sessional consumption: For example, in the United Kingdom, immoderate drinking (above the daily moderate drinking benchmarks of four or three units for men and women, respectively) and binge drinking (more than double these daily benchmarks; i.e., eight or six units for men and women, respectively) by British adults peaked around 2001 and declined slightly thereafter (Goddard, 2006). In the search for new terminology that might encapsulate the key concerns, motivations, and outcomes in relation to contemporary drinking, we have seen the resurrection of the terms *harmful* and *hazardous* drinking from the World Health Organization (WHO), as well as the introduction of the term *extreme drinking* to capture the notion of the pursuit of determined drunkenness (as entertainment despite calculated risk) by some young people (Martinic & Measham, 2008). The terms hazardous and harmful drinking were first employed in a WHO memorandum (Edwards, Arif, & Hodgson, 1981). *Hazardous drinking* refers to a level of consumption or pattern of drinking that, should it persist, is likely to result in harm to the drinker; *harmful drinking* is the next stage, where alcohol consumption has already started to have adverse mental or physical effects but not (yet) alcohol dependency.* The aim of these distinctions is to identify those at-risk individuals who may not yet meet the criteria for alcohol dependence, so that interventions can target them before they have developed chronic alcohol problems that require more intensive interventions.

Such convergence is also in evidence in parts of Asia. In China and Japan, for example, alcohol has been traditionally held in high esteem, and carefully defined drinking etiquettes have governed the circumstances of its intake, with much consumption ritualized in terms of customs such as the order and content of drinks, the ritual and symbolic meaning of rice wine, and the manner of drinking (e.g., reciprocal pouring of drinks and toasting). Historically, not offending one's host has taken precedent over the regulation of intake or the avoidance of excess, leading one anthropologist to note that, in Japan, "It is impolite to be sober when others are not, so newcomers to a party are encouraged to get drunk as soon as possible" (Dalby, 1983, p. 140). Ritualized drunkenness in traditional Japanese society, however, was confined to religious festivals or used to add some levity to otherwise solemn occasions (e.g., work meetings). However, with the changing patterns and societal structure in modern Japan, such unambiguous delineations are disappearing (Sargent, 1979; Schnell, 1997).

Shifts in attitudes toward drunkenness in the last 50 years in both China and Japan show evidence of less excessive drinking during work hours

---

* The terms *hazardous* and *harmful drinking* focus more on weekly consumption, with drinkers exposed to high risk of alcohol-related harm: Hazardous drinkers are defined as men and women whose alcohol intake regularly exceeds recommended sensible levels (in the United Kingdom, over 4 or 3 units per day for men and women, respectively, but, more particularly, over 28 or 21 units per week), and harmful drinkers are defined as those who regularly consume over 8 or 6 units per day (in the United Kingdom, leading to more than 50 or 35 units per week for men and women, respectively—see Department of Health, Home Office, Department for Education and Skills, & Department for Culture, Media and Sport, 2007).

among business associates due to the negative impact on industrial productivity (Hao, Chen, & Su, 2005). The long, alcohol-laden lunches and midday banquets traditionally commonplace among civil servants, for example, are becoming less acceptable due to the dramatic drop in individual productivity that generally follows. An official effort to prevent this practice has been aimed not only at reducing alcohol consumption during work hours, but also at managing expectations and social pressure on individuals to engage in these activities (Yardley, 2008).

This is contrasted with an increasingly favorable attitude toward public drunkenness among young men during leisure time, with the development of a form of male episodic drinking known as "heroic drinking" (Partanen, 2006; see also Martinic & Measham, 2008; Sargent, 1979). The male-dominated nature of drinking venues is still evident in the *sakariba* or drinking zones of Japanese big cities: Employees visit these bars after work to de-stress and informally network with business partners and colleagues, in what the Austrian sociologist Linhart (1986) termed "zones of evaporation," located along major commuter transport routes (p. 206). Women's roles within such drinking establishments tend to be as bar staff, waitresses, and hostesses, paid to serve the predominantly male customer base, and as a small but growing minority of (young) female employees drinking alongside their male colleagues. Drinking is not strictly segregated by gender in Japan, with Smith and Wiswell (1982) noting the bawdy, drunk, and disorderly behavior of women at village weddings and other rural gatherings in both women-only and mixed companies. In urban Japan, however, Hendry (1994) described the continued limited opportunities for women to drink in public space, resulting in the perceived problem of the lonely "kitchen drinker," with an estimated one in four suicides by housewives attributed at least in part to drinking problems (pp. 187–188). Thus, the impact of changing material and sociocultural conditions on the lives of Japanese women and men is evident in changing attitudes toward drunkenness in both public and private spaces.

CONCLUSION

At the heart of this chapter is recognition of the complexities of the experience of drunkenness and of the ambiguities and inconsistencies in attempting to define and measure excessive sessional alcohol consumption. The central challenge is, therefore, to assess prevalence, trends, or outcomes across locality and time, while recognizing that the pleasures of drunkenness as an altered state of intoxication, which people purposefully pursue, remains higher on the agenda of drinkers than researchers. Not only the well-documented pains of this "voluntary madness" but the social and pharmacological pleasures of altered states of intoxication need consideration in developing policy prescriptions that can achieve success.

Official sanction of terms such as binge, harmful, and hazardous drinking has waxed and waned alongside the ebb and flow of new academic terms such as determined drunkenness, calculated hedonism, intense intoxication, and extreme drinking. The continuing importance of not just drinking but drunkenness is evidenced in this evolution of an abundant but disputed terminology to define acute heavy drinking that is of concern to policymakers. This "linguistic friction" illustrates not only the nebulous and problematic nature of the concept of drunkenness, but also, perhaps more important, the fact that the possible pains of this behavior have been subsumed under the "problem" banner *along* with its attendant pleasures. This recent "problematizing" of *all* aspects of drunkenness—the pleasures and the pains—must surely be central to an understanding of modern policy responses.

There are a range of measurements focusing on both the objective state of intoxication (e.g., based on standard drink units, BAC, and the International Classification of Diseases [World Health Organization, 1992] or *Diagnostic and Statistical Manual of Mental Disorders* [4th ed.; American Psychiatric Association, 1994] criteria) and the subjective individual and wider sociocultural experience of drunkenness (e.g., drinkers' own perceptions). For example, unit-based measures of binge drinking have developed to assess the risks of alcohol-related problems, whereas perceptions and experiences of drunkenness have been advocated by some researchers as a more accurate way of predicting harm and tracking cultural shifts in drinking patterns. What is clear is that there is a complex and changing relationship between these more objective measures of alcohol consumption and more subjective perceptions of levels of intoxication, however defined, indicated in the abundance of terms to describe these various states. For some, it is possible to drink within recommended guidelines or at least below unit-based binge-drinking definitions and still feel drunk, particularly for light and occasional drinkers (Midanik, 2003). Others define moderate drinking as not feeling drunk even if they have consumed many more units than public health programs would see as thresholds of moderation (Green et al., 2007). Depending on how intoxication is defined, it is possible to be intoxicated without showing any of the signs commonly associated with drunkenness, particularly among heavier and more frequent drinkers. This questions existing policy responses concerning the framing of alcohol education, information, and interventions when subjective perceptions of drunkenness, sobriety, or cognitive and behavioral functioning may be above or below "official" recommendations. As subjective perceptions might not necessarily relate to either a clear linear relationship or correlation with units of alcohol consumed, drinkers' concerns about the limitations of a "one size fits all" moderate-drinking message seem justified. It also raises the profile of cultural variations in the social norms surrounding drunkenness, reflected, for example, in a historical trend toward the increased identification, treatment, and problematization of drunkenness in the United States (Room, 1991) and the United Kingdom (Measham & Moore, 2008). An interesting point made by Midanik (2003) in her research comparing quantitative and qualitative definitions of drunkenness is that drinkers themselves know when their drunkenness is pleasurable, and, equally, they know when they have had "too much," leading her to conclude that alcohol researchers could perhaps take more notice of drinkers' own judgment.

Whether drunkenness is seen as something to strive for or avoid depends, in part, on academics', policymakers', and drinkers' notions of what drunkenness entails and what they might want to achieve. Although each measurement has its merits and advocates, this chapter concludes that any exploration of contemporary drunkenness reflects the political aims and objectives of a specific investigation. Although Knupfer (1984) suggested that "it is not the *term* that matters: drunkenness itself often has bad *consequences,* which is why we study it" (p. 185, italics in original), this book is testament to a broader perspective—that drunkenness can be a social problem, seen as a measurable risk or a harmful outcome, but it can also be a leisure activity, an individual and social pleasure, a cultural phenomenon, and more, as the following chapter on youth drunkenness explores.

REFERENCES

Alcohol Concern. (2001, January). *Alcohol Concern fact sheet: Alcopops.* Retrieved September 20, 2009, from http://www.alcoholconcern.org.uk/

Alexander, B. (1985). Drug use, dependence and addiction at a British Columbia university: Good news and bad news. *Canadian Journal of Higher Education, 15,* 77–91.

Alexander, B. (2004). A historical analysis of addiction. In P. Rosenqvist, J. Blomqvist, A. Koski-Jannes, & L. Ojesjo (Eds.), *Addiction and life course* (pp. 11–27). Helsinki, Finland: Nordic Council for Alcohol and Drug Research.

American Psychiatric Association. (1994). *The diagnostic and statistical manual of mental disorders* (4th ed.). Washington, DC: American Psychiatric Association.

Babor, T. (1994). Avoiding the horrid and beastly sin of drunkenness: Does dissuasion make a difference? *Journal of Consulting and Clinical Psychology, 62,* 1127–1140.

Baker, A. E. (2003). *A glossary of Northamptonshire words and phrases; with examples of their colloquial use* (Vol. II). London: Cartwright Press. (Original work published 1854)

Barr, A. (1995). *Drink: An informal social history.* London: Bantam.

Bascones Perez-Fragero, A. (2008). *Botellón* in Spain. In M. Martinic & F. Measham (Eds.), *Swimming with crocodiles: The culture of extreme drinking* (pp. 193–197). New York: Routledge.

Bennett, J. M. (1991). Misogyny, popular culture, and women's work. *History Workshop Journal, 31,* 166–188.

Berridge, V. (1981). *Opium and the people: Opiate use and drug control policy in nineteenth and early twentieth century England.* London: Free Association Books.

Borsay, P. (2007, February). *Binge drinking and moral panics: Historical parallels?* Paper presented at the Alcohol Education and Research Council workshop on Addressing Binge Drinking: Challenges and Opportunities, London.

Brain, K., & Parker, H. (1997). *Drinking with design: Alcopops, designer drinks and youth culture.* London: Portman Group.

Brennan, T. E. (1991). Social drinking in Old Regime Paris. In S. Barrows & R. Room (Eds.), *Drinking: Behavior and belief in modern history* (pp. 61–86). Berkeley: University of California Press.

Cameron, D., Thomas, M., Madden, S., Thornton, C., Bergmark, A., Garretsen, H., et al. (2000). Intoxicated across Europe: In search of meaning. *Addiction Research & Theory, 8,* 233–242.

Clark, P. A. (1983). *The English alehouse: A social history 1200–1830.* London: Longman.

Coleman, L., & Cater, S. (2003). What do we know about young people's use of alcohol? *Education and Health, 21,* 50–55.

Coleman, L., & Cater, S. (2005). *Underage "risky" drinking: Motivations and outcomes.* York, UK: Joseph Rowntree Foundation.

Dalby, L. (1983). *Geisha.* Berkeley: University of California Press.

Davies, A. (1992). *Leisure, gender and poverty: Working-class culture in Salford and Manchester, 1900–1939.* Maidenhead, UK: Open University Press.

Davies, J. B. (1997). *The myth of addiction* (2nd ed.). Amsterdam, the Netherlands: Harwood.

Demant, J., & Østergaard, J. (2007). Partying as everyday life: Investigations of teenagers' leisure life. *Journal of Youth Studies, 10,* 517–537.

Department of Health, Home Office, Department for Education and Skills, & Department for Culture, Media and Sport. (2007). *Safe. Sensible. Social. The next steps in the National Alcohol Strategy.* London: The Stationery Office.

Douglas, M. (1987). A distinctive anthropological perspective. In M. Douglas (Ed.), *Constructive drinking: Perspectives on drink from anthropology* (pp. 3–15). Cambridge, UK: Cambridge University Press.

Dunstan, K. (1968). *Wowsers.* Melbourne, Australia: Cassell.

Edwards, G., Arif, A., & Hodgson, R. (1981). Nomenclature and classification of drug- and alcohol-related problems: A WHO memorandum. *Bulletin of the World Health Organization, 59,* 225–242.

El-Guebaly, N., & El-Guebaly, A. (1981). Alcohol abuse in ancient Egypt: The recorded evidence. *Substance Use & Misuse, 16,* 1207–1221.

Ettorre, E. (1997). *Women & alcohol: A private pleasure or a public problem?* London: Women's Press.

Featherstone, M. (1991). *Consumer culture and postmodernity.* London: Sage.

Forsyth, A. (2001). A design for strife: Alcopops, licit drug—Familiar scare story. *International Journal of Drug Policy, 12,* 59–80.

Foster, P. (1995). *Women and the health care industry: An unhealthy relationship?* Buckingham, UK: Open University Press.

Gefou-Madianou, D. (Ed.). (1992). *Alcohol, gender and culture.* London: Routledge.

Goddard, E. (2006, November). *General household survey 2005: Smoking and drinking among adults, 2005.* London: Office for National Statistics.

Goddard, E. (2007, December). *Estimating alcohol consumption from survey data: Updated method of converting volumes to units* (National Statistics Methodological Series No. 37). Newport, UK: Office for National Statistics.

Goddard, E., & Green, H. (2005). *General household survey 2004: Smoking and drinking among adults, 2004.* London: Office for National Statistics.

Gollancz, V. (1972). *Mass observation: The pub and the people.* London: Seven Dials Press. (Original work published 1943)

Green, C., Polen, M., Janoff, S., Castleton, D., & Perrin, N. (2007). "Not getting tanked": Definitions of moderate drinking and their health implications. *Drug and Alcohol Dependence, 86,* 265–273.

Gusfield, J. (1986). *Symbolic crusade: Status politics and the American temperance movement* (2nd ed.). Champaign: University of Illinois Press.

Hadfield, P. (Ed.). (2009). *Nightlife and crime.* Oxford, UK: Oxford University Press.

Hao, W., Chen, H., & Su, Z. (2005). China: Alcohol today. *Addiction, 100,* 737–741.

Harrison, B. (1971). *Drink and the Victorians: The temperance question in England 1815–1872.* Pittsburgh, PA: University of Pittsburgh Press.

Hayward, K., & Hobbs, D. (2007). Beyond the binge in "booze Britain": Market-led liminalization and the spectacle of binge drinking. *British Journal of Sociology, 58,* 437–456.

Heath, D. B. (2000). *Drinking occasions: Comparative perspectives on alcohol and culture.* Philadelphia: Brunner/Mazel.

Hendry, J. (1994). Drinking and gender in Japan. In M. McDonald (Ed.), *Gender, drink and drugs* (pp. 175–190). Oxford, UK: Berg.

Herring, R., Berridge, V., & Thom, B. (2008). Binge drinking: An exploration of a confused concept. *Journal of Epidemiology and Community Health, 62,* 476–479.

Hibell, B., Andersson, B., Bjarnason, T., Ahlström, S., Balakireva, O., Kokkevi, A., et al. (2004). *The ESPAD report 2003: Alcohol and other drug use among students in 35 European countries.* Stockholm: The Swedish Council for Information on Alcohol and Other Drugs.

Hibell, B., Guttormsson, U., Ahlström, S., Balakireva, O., Bjarnason, T., Kokkevi, A., et al. (2009). *The 2007 ESPAD report: Substance use among students in 35 European countries.* Stockholm: The Swedish Council for Information on Alcohol and Other Drugs.

Hitting the drink. (2008, June 15). *The Sunday Age,* pp. 15–16.

Horne, D. (1964). *The lucky country: Australia in the sixties.* Melbourne, Australia: Penguin Books.

Horton, D. J. (1943). The function of alcohol in primitive societies: A cross-cultural study. *Quarterly Journal of Studies on Alcohol, 4,* 199–320.

Hughes, K., Anderson, Z., Morleo, M., & Bellis, M. A. (2007). Alcohol, nightlife and violence: The relative contributions of drinking before and during nights out to negative health and criminal justice outcomes. *Addiction, 103,* 60–65.

Jackson, C., & Tinkler, P. (2007). "Ladettes" and "modern girls": "Troublesome" young femininities. *Sociological Review, 55,* 251–272.

James, O. (2007). *Affluenza.* London: Vermillion.

James, O. (2008). *The selfish capitalist: Origins of affluenza.* London: Vermilion.

Jarvinen, M., & Room, R. (Eds.). (2007). *Youth drinking cultures: European experiences.* Farnham, UK: Ashgate.

Jayne, M., Valentine, G., & Holloway, S. L. (2008). Fluid boundaries—British binge drinking and European civility: Alcohol and the production and consumption of public space. *Space and Polity, 12,* 81–100.

Jellinek, E. M. (1976). Drinkers and alcoholics in ancient Rome. *Journal of Studies on Alcohol, 37,* 1718–1741.

Kilmer, J. R., & Larimer, M. E. (2008). Case study: Drinking among sorority and fraternity students in the United States. In M. Martinic & F. Measham (Eds.), *Swimming with crocodiles: The culture of extreme drinking* (pp. 228–232). New York: Routledge.

Kirkby, D. (2003). Beer, glorious beer: Gender politics and Australian popular culture. *Journal of Popular Culture, 37,* 244–256.

Knupfer, G. (1984). The risks of drunkenness (or, *ebrietas resurrecta*): A comparison of frequent intoxication indices and of population sub-groups as to problem risks. *British Journal of Addiction, 79,* 185–196.

Kohn, M. (1992). *Dope girls: The birth of the British drug underground.* London: Lawrence & Wishart.

Kohn, M. (1997). The chemical generation and its ancestors: Dance crazes and drug panics across eight decades. *International Journal of Drug Policy, 8,* 137–142.

Leigh, B. C. (1984). *1984 Drinking Attitudes Study* [Unpublished data]. Berkeley, CA: Alcohol Research Group.

Levine, H. G. (1978). The discovery of addiction: Changing conceptions of habitual drunkenness in America. *Journal of Studies on Alcohol, 39,* 143–174.

Levine, H. G. (1981). The vocabulary of drunkenness. *Journal of Studies on Alcohol, 42,* 1038–1051.

Levine, H. G. (1984). The alcohol problem in America: From temperance to alcoholism. *British Journal of Addiction, 79,* 109–119.

Lewis, M. (1992). *A rum state: Alcohol and state policy in Australia, 1788–1988.* Canberra: Australian Government Publishing Service.

Lewis, M. (2006). *Alcohol in Australia: The intertwining of social and personal histories: An interview with Milton Lewis.* Retrieved September 20, 2009, from http://www.dulwichcentre.com.au/alcohol_in_australia.htm (Original work published 1997)

Linhart, S. (1986). Sakariba: Zone of "evaporation" between work and home? In J. Hendry & J. Webber (Eds.), *Interpreting Japanese society: Anthropological approaches* (pp. 231–242). Oxford, UK: Oxford University Press.

Luckins, T. (2007). Pigs, hogs and Aussie blokes: The emergence of the term "six o'clock swill." *History Australia, 4,* 1–17.

MacAndrew, C., & Edgerton, R. C. (2003). *Drunken comportment: A social explanation.* Clinton Corners, NY: Percheron Press/Eliot Werner Publications. (Original work published 1969)

Martinic, M., & Measham, F. (Eds.). (2008). *Swimming with crocodiles: The culture of extreme drinking.* New York: Routledge.

McCandless, P. (1984). "Curses of civilization": Insanity and drunkenness in Victorian Britain. *British Journal of Addiction, 79,* 49–58.

McDonald, M. (1994). Drinking and social identity in the west of France. In M. McDonald (Ed.), *Gender, drink and drugs* (pp. 99–124). Oxford, UK: Berg.

McKeganey, N. (1998). Alcopops and young people: A suitable cause for concern. *Addiction, 93,* 471–473.

McKeganey, N., Forsyth, A., Barnard, M., & Hay, G. (1996). Designer drinks and drunkenness amongst a sample of Scottish schoolchildren. *British Medical Journal, 313,* 401.

Measham, F. (2002). "Doing gender"—"doing drugs": Conceptualising the gendering of drug cultures. *Contemporary Drug Problems, 29,* 335–373.

Measham, F. (2006). The new policy mix: Alcohol, harm minimisation and determined drunkenness in contemporary society. *International Journal of Drug Policy, 17,* 258–268.

Measham, F. (2008). A history of intoxication: Changing attitudes to drunkenness and excess in the United Kingdom. In M. Martinic & F. Measham (Eds.), *Swimming with crocodiles: The culture of extreme drinking* (pp. 13–36). New York: Routledge.

Measham, F., & Brain, K. (2005). "Binge" drinking, British alcohol policy and the new culture of intoxication. *Crime, Media, Culture: An International Journal, 1,* 262–283.

Measham, F., & Moore, K. (2008). The criminalisation of intoxication. In P. Squires (Ed.), *ASBO nation: The criminalisation of nuisance* (pp. 273–288). Bristol, UK: Policy.

Measham, F., & Østergaard, J. (2009). The public face of binge drinking: British and Danish young women, recent trends in alcohol consumption and the European binge drinking debate. *Probation Journal, 56,* 415–434.

Midanik, L. T. (1999). Drunkenness, feeling the effects and 5 plus measures. *Addiction, 94,* 887–897.

Midanik, L. T. (2003). Definitions of drunkenness. *Substance Use and Misuse, 38,* 1285–1303.

Ngokwey, N. (1987). Varieties of palm wine among the Lele of the Kasai. In M. Douglas (Ed.), *Constructive drinking: Perspectives on drink from anthropology* (pp. 113–121). Cambridge, UK: Cambridge University Press.

Parker, H., Aldridge, J., & Measham, F. (1998). *Illegal leisure: The normalization of adolescent recreational drug use among English youth.* London: Routledge.

Parker, H., & Williams, L. (2003). Intoxicated weekends: Young adults' work hard–play hard lifestyles, public health and public disorder. *Drugs: Education, Prevention, and Policy, 10,* 345–367.

Partanen, J. (2006). Spectacles of sociability and drunkenness: On alcohol and drinking in Japan. *Contemporary Drug Problems, 33,* 177–204.
Pearson, G. (1983). *Hooligan: A history of respectable fears.* Basingstoke, UK: Macmillan.
Plant, M. (1997). *Women and alcohol: Contemporary and historical perspectives.* London: Free Association Books.
Plant, M., & Plant, M. (2006). *Binge Britain: Alcohol and the national response.* Oxford, UK: Oxford University Press.
Porter, R. (1985). The drinking man's disease: The "pre-history" of alcoholism in Georgian Britain. *Addiction, 80,* 385–396.
Presdee, M. (2000). *Cultural criminology and the carnival of crime.* London: Routledge.
Richardson, A., & Budd, T. (2003). *Alcohol, crime and disorder: A study of young adults* (Home Office Research Study 263). London: Home Office.
Roche, A. M., Bywood, P. T., Borlagdan, J., Lunnay, B., Freeman, T., Lawton, L., et al. (2007). *Young people and alcohol: The role of cultural influences.* Adelaide, Australia: National Centre for Education and Training on Addiction.
Room, R. (1988). The dialectic of drinking in Australian life: From the rum corps to the wine column. *Australian Drug and Alcohol Review, 7,* 413–437.
Room, R. (1991). Cultural changes in drinking and trends in alcohol problems indicators: Recent U.S. experience. In W. Clark & M. Hilton (Eds.), *Alcohol in America: Drinking practices and problems in a national survey* (pp. 149–162). Albany: State University of New York Press.
Room, R. (2005). Multicultural contexts and alcohol and drug use as symbolic behaviour. *Addiction Research & Theory, 13,* 321–331.
Rosovsky, H. (1999). Drinking and pleasure in Latin America. In S. Peele & M. Grant (Eds.), *Alcohol and pleasure* (pp. 87–100). Philadelphia: Brunner/Mazel.
Sargent, M. J. (1979). Changes in Japanese drinking patterns. In M. Marshall (Ed.), *Beliefs, behaviors, and alcoholic beverages* (pp. 278–288). Ann Arbor: University of Michigan Press.
Schnell, S. (1997). Sanctity and sanction in communal ritual: A reconsideration of Shint festival processions. *Ethnology, 36,* 1–12.
Schuckit, M. A. (1998). The editor responds. *Journal of Studies on Alcohol, 59,* 123–124.
Segal, B. M. (1986). The Soviet heavy-drinking culture and the American heavy-drinking subculture. *Annals of the New York Academy of Sciences, 472,* 149–160.
Smith, R. J., & Wiswell, E. L. (1982). *The women of Suye Mura.* Chicago: University of Chicago Press.
Social Issues Research Centre. (1998). *Social and cultural aspects of drinking.* Oxford, UK: Author.
Squires, P. (Ed.). (2008). *ASBO nation: The criminalisation of nuisance.* Bristol, UK: Policy.
Stockley, C. S. (1998). The safe use of alcohol during pregnancy. *International Journal of Drug Policy, 9,* 273–276.
Stockwell, T., Rydon, P., Gianatti, S., Jenkins, E., Ovenden, C., & Syed, D. (1992). Levels of drunkenness of customers leaving licensed premises in Perth, Western Australia: A comparison of high and low "risk" premises. *British Journal of Addiction, 87,* 873–881.
Szmigin, I., Griffin, C., Mistral, W., Bengry-Howell, A., Weale, L., & Hackley, C. (2008). Re-framing "binge drinking" as calculated hedonism: Empirical evidence from the U.K. *International Journal of Drug Policy, 19,* 359–366.

Thombs, D., Dodd, V., Pokorny, S., Omli, M. R., O'Mara, R., Webb, M. C., et al. (2008). Drink specials and the intoxication levels of patrons exiting college bars. *American Journal of Health Behavior, 32,* 411–419.

Tuck, M. (1989). *Drinking and disorder: A study of non-metropolitan violence.* London: Stationery Office Books.

Warner, J. (1997). The sanctuary of sobriety: The emergence of temperance as a feminine virtue in Tudor and Stuart England. *Addiction, 92,* 97–111.

Warner, J. (2003). *Craze: Gin and debauchery in an age of reason.* London: Random House Trade Paperbacks.

Wechsler, H., Davenport, A., Dowdall, G., Moeykens, B., & Castillo, S. (1994). Health and behavioral consequences of binge drinking in college: A national survey of students at 140 campuses. *Journal of the American Medical Association, 272,* 1672–1677.

Wechsler, H., Dowdall, G., Davenport, A., & Castillo, S. (1995). Correlates of college student binge drinking. *American Journal of Public Health, 85,* 921–926.

Wechsler, H., & Isaac, N. (1992). "Binge" drinkers at Massachusetts colleges: Prevalence, drinking style, time trends, and associated problems. *Journal of the American Medical Association, 267,* 2929–2931.

Wechsler, H., Kuh, G., & Davenport, A. (1996). Fraternities, sororities and binge drinking: Results from a national study of American colleges. *NASPA Journal, 33,* 260–279.

Williams, G. P., & Brake, G. T. (1980). *Drink in Great Britain, 1900–1979.* London: Edsall.

World Health Organization. (1992). *The ICD-10 classification of mental and behavioural disorders: Clinical descriptions and diagnostic guidelines.* Geneva, Switzerland: Author.

Yardley, J. (2008, March 8). Got a mint, comrade? Chinese ban liquid lunch. *The New York Times* (Online). Retrieved September 9, 2009, from http://www.nytimes.com/2008/03/08/world/asia/08china.html

Zinberg, N. E. (1984). *Drug, set, and setting: The basis for controlled intoxicant use.* New Haven, CT: Yale University Press.

5

Drinking Contexts and Youth Drunkenness

Betsy Thom, with Irmgard Eisenbach-Stangl

This chapter examines how youth drunkenness is shaped and constrained by social and cultural forces in contemporary drinking contexts. Our focus here is on young people under 25 years old, which includes both young adults and underage drinkers.* In previous chapters, we saw that how people think about drunkenness, how they behave when drunk, and the extent to which drunkenness and different degrees of drunkenness are tolerated are historically, culturally, and socially defined. We have also seen that factors such as age, gender, social status, ethnicity, and religion are important influences on how people drink and behave around alcohol. Equally, in most societies we find formal and informal regulatory systems, customs, and traditions setting normative boundaries on alcohol consumption, drunkenness, and related behaviors. Such "cultural universals" are a feature of all societies where alcohol is consumed, but the forms in which they appear differ greatly from place to place (Heath, 2000; Järvinen & Room, 2007). Even today when, according to some accounts, mass communication, travel, and global marketing have resulted in a considerable degree of lifestyle convergence (especially in aspirations for Western lifestyles), there remains a wide diversity of national and local attitudes and responses toward drunkenness and numerous ways in which different social groups display it (Beccaria & Sande, 2003). In contrast to early societies where drinking

* Most countries where alcohol consumption is legal have a mandated threshold age at which buying and consuming alcohol becomes permitted, ranging from 16 to 25 years of age, with 18 being the most common age limit. Where the age limit is set, it is largely a product of cultural attitudes toward alcohol and level of permissiveness toward drinking by young people. Typically, drinking age laws make no reference to alcohol consumption in the home. In some countries, alcohol content or type of beverage also determines the age of legal access. For a table listing minimum age limits in a number of countries around the world, see www.icap.org/table/MinimumAgeLimitsWorldwide

behaviors were determined largely by the immediate family, community, or social group, behavior in the modern world is influenced by much wider national and global forces, as well as by the more localized situations and specific cultural contexts of everyday life.

We begin with the drinking context as a framework for drunkenness and consider the argument that drunkenness is linked to and reflects wider national characteristics. The regulations governing access to alcohol and the nature of the drinking environment—both indoor and outdoor—likely set the parameters that define acceptable and unacceptable consumption levels and conduct for the society as a whole. The chapter continues with a discussion of the more immediate factors within the drinking environment that have been found to influence youth drunkenness. Contributions from the perspective of social geography have recently highlighted how social space, its management, and "ownership" by different groups influence behavior (Jayne, Valentine, & Holloway, 2008c).

We then address the normative context of drunkenness. Research has shown that beliefs about how others drink have a part to play in one's choices about alcohol. There are numerous occasions when drunken behaviors are socially permissible—at least to some degree for those whose age permits them to drink; at the individual level, life transitions (e.g., births, marriages, and deaths) and, at the community level, public festivities (e.g., Mardi Gras carnivals in Brazil) are events when the everyday barriers on behavior are lowered (Heath, 2000). Alcohol and drunkenness are often constant features of such ceremonial occasions, and it is the enduring beliefs about the role of alcohol within ritual practices (whether modern or "traditional") that function as factors in either encouraging or tolerating drunken behavior for some people under some circumstances. As an example, we draw on studies of young people's drinking that examine the meaning and function of drunkenness as a part of modern rites of passage (e.g., school graduation and university entrance) and the negotiation or renegotiation of identity and position within social groups.

However, drunken behavior is both shaped by and, in turn, helps to shape social responses. Examples are provided from research undertaken in two countries, Austria and Scotland, to show how similar levels or types of drunken behavior can elicit very different responses depending on such factors as the age, gender, or socioeconomic status of the drinker or the cultural and social context within which drunkenness occurs. In these studies, differences in policing procedures and professional interventions toward different groups of young people display the application of variable, "elastic" normative responses.

This chapter focuses on young people because they are often seen as most prone to public displays of drunkenness, and they are the group that has attracted the greatest professional, media, and policy attention, as demonstrated by Case Study 5.1 on the British experience at the end of the chapter. It is in looking at young people that we can begin to address current questions about possible generational shifts in drinking cultures, cultures of drunkenness, and factors related to change. The new youthful drinking patterns have been observed over a number of years in many European countries—for instance, in Spain (Rodrigues-Martos, 2006) and the United Kingdom (see Parker, Aldridge, & Measham, 1998), as well as in Austria, where it is discussed under the pejorative heading of *Komatrinken,* or *coma drinking* (Sadounig, 2008). The perceived trend toward more young people becoming involved in unacceptable drunken behaviors was voiced in the World Health Organization's *Declaration on Young People and Alcohol,* which stated that:

> The main trends in the drinking patterns of young people are greater experimentation with alcohol among children and increases in high-risk drinking patterns such as "binge drinking" and drunkenness, especially among adolescents and young adults. (World Health Organization Regional Office for Europe, 2001, para. 4)

It is important, therefore, to consider the factors that influence young people's drinking and the social and normative contexts (beyond alcohol policy approaches) that serve to sustain or restrain their drunkenness.

THE SOCIAL CONTEXT OF DRUNKENNESS

The Indoor Drinking Environment

The design and management of the indoor drinking environment have been the focus of research in several countries, generating a considerable list of features seen as likely to prevent or ameliorate drinking, drunkenness, and other unacceptable behavior—and of those that have the opposite effect of increasing their likelihood. Some of the earliest work looking at ways of preventing aggression in barroom settings highlighted both the physical environment and the environment of social control within venues (reviewed in Graham & Homel, 1997). Design features such as comfort, roominess, ventilation, and how well-kept and attractive the premises are have been found to influence customers' expectations about the establishment and its management. At the same time, the relationship between design features and drunkenness is not clear cut. Graham and Homel (1997) provided the example of a respectable bar in Texas where shabby, poorly maintained premises were a deliberate part of the décor, a demonstration of resistance to trends toward "yuppy" bars (p. 174). Nevertheless, there is a general consensus in the literature that drunkenness and aggression tend to be associated with poor ventilation, lack of adequate seating, high noise levels, low levels of lighting, difficult access to the bar and toilets, and other environmental factors that may irritate or frustrate patrons (Graham & Homel, 1997, 2008; Hadfield, 2006).

The development of giant "vertical drinking establishments"—crowded, noisy, and incorporating many of the design features likely to increase drunkenness and bad behavior—was one of the factors picked out by the critics of the 2003 Alcohol Licensing Act in England and Wales (The Stationery Office, 2003, 2005) and has been described in studies of the nighttime economy. In one account, a bar owner estimated that around 3,500 to 4,000 people entered his establishment on a Saturday night, which meant around 8,000 journeys up and down a narrow entrance staircase, a "big flashpoint" for that particular venue (Hadfield, 2006, p. 84). The problems encountered in large drinking venues in the United Kingdom were also acknowledged at the government level and linked to concerns over binge drinking among young people:

> The context in which [binge drinking] takes place also deserves attention. Bars designed to offer drinking while standing as the only entertaining activity ("vertical drinking establishments") and irresponsible promotions such as happy hours, "two for the price of one" and "all you can drink for £10" are thought to contribute to [binge drinking] among young people. (Parliamentary Office of Science and Technology, 2005, p. 2)

This quotation underlines the importance of other elements influencing drunken behavior in indoor public settings: the social ambience of the drinking context and the ways in which patrons are managed and controlled. According to Graham and Homel (1997), these factors are even more central to alcohol-related behavior than the physical design of premises.

Although there are many typologies of drinking establishments, drawing attention to the diversity of such venues, their clientele, and drinking patterns (Graham & Homel, 2008, p. 18), commentators frequently resort to contrasting large modern corporate premises with the more traditional pub. In the traditional English public house, displays of drunken behavior were controlled in numerous subtle ways: Publicans were often respected authority figures embedded in the social life of their communities. In small communities where most people knew each other, fear of getting a "bad reputation" placed boundaries on unacceptable behavior. In working-class industrial areas, bars tended to be largely male preserves where older men passed on the "rules" of drinking and drinking comportment to their siblings, sons, and younger men (Hadfield, 2006, pp. 85–86). Although the form may have changed, there is still a perception, particularly within rural areas, of the village pub as a place at the center of community life, where identities are forged and social standing claimed, and where drinking is controlled by feelings of belonging and aspiration (Heley, 2008).

The idealized picture of the traditional rural pub with its system of mainly informal checks and balances on unacceptable public drunkenness contrasts sharply with observational accounts of establishments where there are large numbers of patrons who are not known to each other or the staff, where staff turnover may be high, and where patrons are likely to be predominantly young. In the latter setting, greater permissiveness regarding swearing and rowdy behavior, sexual activity, competitive games, sale of illegal drugs, availability (or lack) of food, the degree of hostility (or friendliness) shown to strangers, and the ways in which bar staff and security deal with patrons are some of the factors that create the ambiance and influence the occurrence of problematic behavior or serve to maintain peace (Graham & Homel, 2008). In such a setting, more formal regulatory structures and processes, such as server training, are put in place in attempts to manage the clientele. An example of a well-known project in Australia illustrates the importance of the drinking environment and demonstrates both the potential and the limitations of modern control systems.

The Surfers Paradise prevention program on the Queensland Gold Coast, a tourist area with large numbers of transient young people, was intended to reduce violence, crime, and disorder associated with drunkenness in and around licensed premises. Using approaches such as risk assessments in drinking establishments, promotion of a code of practice, and monitoring by police and licensing officials to enforce refusal of alcohol to intoxicated patrons, the project enjoyed considerable short-term success in changing the drinking environment and ameliorating problems. Unfortunately, longer term follow-up revealed the fragility of the changes: There had been a temporary displacement of drunk and disorderly clients to adjoining areas; after the project ended, they returned to Surfers Paradise, and violence rose again to preproject levels (Midford, Wayte, Catalano, Gupta, & Chikritzhs, 2005). This example illustrates the difficulties of controlling youth drunken behavior through authorities external to the social group, whereby such initiatives can only succeed with constant, and perhaps costly, vigilance. Contrast this with the traditional pub and its more sustainable system of mainly informal checks and balances on unacceptable public drunkenness by the more mature members of the social group.

The Outdoor Drinking Environment

Trouble in the streets may well be linked to incidents that happen inside premises, as angry or frustrated patrons are ejected from venues, refused alcohol, or find themselves jostling at fast-food restaurants or taxi stands. There are numerous accounts of the importance of public space, its contested "ownership" and symbolic value as a "stage" where youthful carnivalesque (and usually drunken) behavior is performed, and of attempts to constrain and control behavior in public places (Jayne, Valentine, & Holloway, 2008a, 2008c). As Graham and Homel (2008) argued, street drunkenness, especially in areas with a concentration of youth nightlife, has become a political issue in many countries (see Case Study 5.1 at the end of this chapter).

The Bigg Market area of Newcastle typifies the city center leisure drinking environment described in U.K. studies. The special buzz and lively atmosphere of the Bigg Market derives as much from what happens on the streets as in the bars themselves. Chatterton and Hollands (2001) described the

> large, "vertical drinking" fun pubs and "disco bars" . . . based around loud music, cheap drinks, happy hours, open spaces with few seats and a high turnover of consumers. The intimate and dense networks of such pubs stretching across a tightly bound labyrinth of cobbled streets, creates a stage between these pubs for roving groups of lads and lasses. (p. 75)

The authors proposed that drunkenness was the inevitable outcome of the "circuit drinking" that intimidates some people who do not feel part of the roving, rowdy groups and invigorates the "insiders" who feel "really powerful in a horrible sort of way . . . it's like you own the city" (Chatterton & Hollands, 2001, p. 75).

Graham and Homel (2008) proposed a number of ways in which alcohol-related aggression outside is linked to specific licensed premises: entry practices that are seen as unfair or confrontational, clashes between groups coming out of different premises, ejection of troublesome patrons, aggression between ejected patrons and staff, movement between establishments (e.g., the "circuit drinking" in the Bigg Market), and crowds watching and sometimes participating in conflicts (Graham & Homel, 2008, p. 170). Although density of venues within an area will not necessarily result in problems, it appears to be an important factor in shaping alcohol-related behaviors in some U.K. inner cities (Graham & Homel, 2008, p. 178).

However, factors other than density have also been seen as exacerbating or reducing unwelcome drunkenness. Attempts to address related problems in three British cities—Birmingham, Cardiff, and Glasgow—included both on-premise interventions such as server training and modifications to the outdoor settings in and around premises. Improved street lighting, use of closed-circuit television, visible policing, and better late-night taxi and bus services were reported to reduce the incidence of violence and nuisance associated with drinking in the targeted areas (Mastache, Mistral, Velleman, & Templeton, 2008; Mistral, Velleman, Mastache, & Templeton, 2007).

The relationship between this new form of urban, leisure-based youth activity and drinking is not confined to the United Kingdom. Describing the emergence of the *botellón* phenomenon in Spain, Gómez Fraguela, Fernández Pérez, Romero Triñanes, and Luengo Martín (2008) reported changes in traditional drinking patterns of young people, related, among other things, to the reinvention and youthful acquisition of public space, a pattern of heavy weekend consumption, and a rise in city center problems similar to those reported in U.K. studies. The authors maintained that, since the phenomenon was first observed in 1995, it has spread to most Spanish cities. However, it is mainly younger adolescents who become involved in the scene, due partly to peer influence and partly to easier availability of alcohol in unsupervised settings than at licensed premises. In this respect, *botellón* may be more akin to underage drinking in public areas than the nighttime economy scenes described earlier. Coleman and Cater (2005), in a U.K. survey of 14- to 17-year-olds with experience of excessive single-session alcohol consumption in unsupervised environments, reported that, although the respondents were aware of the dangers involved and adopted strategies to manage them, most said they enjoyed "risky" drinking patterns. As in other studies, "pushing the boundaries" and achieving a sense of being invincible were as important to drinkers as having fun, easing social interaction, or achieving unexpected loss of control (Coleman & Cater, 2005; see also Galloway, Forsyth, & Shewan, 2007; Harnett, Thom, Herring, & Kelly, 2000; Martinic & Measham, 2008). For some groups of young people, exclusion from the adult drinking environments was one of the factors that facilitated the creation of an alternative culture in which alcohol played an important role.

An examination of youth cultures and the circumstances under which drunkenness is engaged in, tolerated, or frowned on illustrates many of the ways in which behavior is shaped in the modern world. Not least, the literature points to the need to take into account the dynamics of this process, viewing individuals and groups as actors creating the social and normative boundaries of behavior and not merely reacting to the rules, sanctions, and limits placed on them. This brings to the fore differences between subgroups of young people and the ways in which the normative context that shapes drunkenness is itself subject to the variable perceptions and actions of authority figures, professionals, the media, and other social groups, frequently based on factors such as socioeconomic status, fashions, and lifestyles.

THE NORMATIVE CONTEXT OF DRUNKENNESS

Permissible Drunkenness

In some contexts, drunkenness can be understood as a purposeful and managed behavior, for instance, symbolizing transition from one social status to another, providing "time out" from everyday responsibilities or a way of having a socially sanctioned "moral holiday" (as during a *fiesta*), and demonstrating shared experiences with a peer group. The factors that influence drinking patterns on such occasions can take the form of formal rules agreed on by the group or can be informal and unspoken but nevertheless operate to provide boundaries and restrain unacceptable drunken behaviors. These rules set the normative context within which drunkenness is formed and contained. Drinking games, common to most countries, exemplify the situation where drunkenness is allowed and may even be the main aim of the occasion, but the behavior is shaped and bounded by group rules concerning who drinks, when, and how much (Beccaria & Sande, 2003). In many countries, school graduation parties and university entrance celebrations are also occasions when there tends to be an assumption by participants that getting drunk will be an outcome of the event. Drunkenness may be accompanied by more or less formalized ways of behaving, symbolically important for participants and grounded in the norms and traditions of the particular group or institution.

The Norwegian Russefeiring

The *russefeiring* tradition in Norway, which began as an elite initiation rite for students at the University of Oslo, has become an integral part of youth culture as a graduation party for young people leaving upper secondary school. It consists of 17 days of celebration, drunkenness, and rule breaking, ending on the Norwegian National Day, May 17. Elected student committees, composed of the upcoming school graduates, make decisions about planned activities and the credits awarded for particular transgressions. Students wear a red *russe* cap, and rule breaking is symbolized by the trophies hanging on the tail of the cap: For example, drinking 24 bottles of beer during a period of 24 hours is rewarded with a beer cork, a jelly candy is given for kissing a policeman, and a liquor cork is the prize for drinking a whole bottle of spirits in 24 hours. There is competition to gain the most trophies for rule breaking, and the winners are honored by the committees. The high points of the celebration, involving heavy drinking and drunkenness, take place on weekends and especially on the night before May 17, when new school graduates participate in large regional outdoor rock music festivals. As part of the tradition, young people have constructed their own system of self-regulation and defined their own behavioral norms with regard to breaking public law and order; parents, police, and other adults accept and tolerate the ensuing drunkenness and violation of rules. (This account has been summarized from Beccaria & Sande, 2003.)

In their analysis of the Norwegian *russefeiring* and similar rites of passage elsewhere, Beccaria and Sande (2003) suggested that during the ceremonial process young people enter what van Gennep (1909/2004) in his seminal work *The Rites of Passage* referred to as a *liminal phase*—outside everyday social structure, roles, and categories, where the behavioral norms stress fun, carnival, partying, and celebration. Drunkenness can be understood as part of this process of transition, which first places young people outside normal social boundaries for behavior and then leads to a new phase of integration into the social structure through the acquisition of a new identity and status. When the factors influencing youth drunkenness are linked to the transitional process, bounded by time, space, and the (alternative) rule-governed transition function, the displays of drunkenness and rule breaking do not constitute a threat to dominant normative behavior (see Chapter 3).

On the other hand, youth drunkenness rituals could also be interpreted as revealing new forms of social differentiation and cultural innovation, especially within or linked to youth cultures in modern societies. From this perspective, the centrality of drunkenness and associated rule breaking in some youth cultures may be seen as a threat to older generations and to "traditional" norms and behavioral patterns. Jayne, Valentine, and Holloway (2008b) suggested that adolescents and young adults often become the centers of public controversies and the targets of repressive regulatory rhetoric when questions of blame and responsibility arise. Panic dynamics, they argued, tend to refocus controversies on youth transgressions as debates about risks get reframed within the policy options for regulation. Media reports on so-called binge drinking (see discussion in Chapter 4), for instance, tend to focus on the threatening, destructive elements of drunkenness, regarding the behavior as unbounded and unmanaged rather than a more transient phase, whether it is a transition from the work week to leisure or from one social status to another (e.g., the Norwegian *russefeiring*). Thus, normative contexts that are tolerant of drunkenness are subject to perceptions of the meaning of the drunken behavior or the degree to which the behavior or the group involved appears hostile to prevailing beliefs and approaches to drunkenness (see discussion in Thom, 2007). This, in turn, is reflected in different reactions and responses to similar degrees of drunkenness or types of alcohol-related behavior.

Permissible Drunkenness: All Is Not Equal

The laws governing youthful alcohol consumption could be seen, therefore, to illustrate the view that regulations on drinking and intoxication reflect societal rejection of and hostility against particular behaviors within certain population subgroups displaying them, as well as concerns to protect vulnerable groups and individuals (Eisenbach-Stangl, Bernardis, Fellöcker, Haberhauer-Stidl, & Schmied, 2008; Uhl & Kobrna, 2008; see Case Study 2.1 in Chapter 2). However, in the preceding sections, we have already seen how behaviors regarded at some times and in some places as unacceptable are tolerated or even encouraged at other times and within different social contexts. Furthermore, within the more uniform picture of regulation on youthful drinking, studies have found considerable variation in the permission granted to different social groups regarding becoming drunk and their conduct when drunk. For example, research on youthful drinking scenes in Vienna and Lower Austria (Eisenbach-Stangl et al., 2008) and in Scotland (Galloway et al., 2007) provided an interesting insight into how drunkenness is linked to social contexts and the different opportunities, circumstances, and lifestyles of individuals and subcultures, and how it is, at least partly, a result of social responses—public and professional perceptions of different groups, their cultures, and activities. The hostility or suspicion shown toward some groups rather than others is illustrated in the following accounts.

Youth Drunkenness Scenes in Vienna and Lower Austria

A study was carried out in the Austrian capital city, Vienna, and in provincial and rural areas in Lower Austria, the state surrounding Vienna

(Eisenbach-Stangl et al., 2008). About 100 key informant interviews were conducted with professionals familiar with young people's drinking; these included street workers, police, nightclub owners, petrol station and convenience store attendants, and private security guards. The interviews were used to construct a number of typical *youth alcohol scenes,* as they were called to acknowledge the arenas or "stages" the young people often chose as settings for their drinking. More than 70 nonparticipant observations of selected youth alcohol scenes were undertaken. The observations, lasting between 30 minutes and 4 hours, concentrated on young people's behaviors but also covered the groups of adults present in the respective settings and their activities. The research yielded information on both youthful drinking and drunkenness and the possible influence of different types of stakeholders and their (re)actions to youthful behavior. Three typical alcohol scenes were identified: the *street scene,* the *disco scene,* and the *private scene.* The private scene had much in common with the *russefeiring* events described earlier, but the other two scenes attracted public disapproval and were subject to intervention from control agencies.

The Street Scene

The most visible and, presumably, the oldest type of youth alcohol scene described by Eisenbach-Stangl and colleagues (2008) was the street scene, involving young people drinking on the streets and in parks, shopping malls, and courtyards of apartment houses, some occasionally engaging in heavy drinking, fighting, and vandalism. The participants of street scenes mostly came from low socioeconomic backgrounds; they were short of money and could not afford to visit pubs or nightclubs. These youths were also the youngest, with a considerable percentage under 16 years old and, therefore, not allowed to drink in pubs or clubs in many countries (including Austria). Public drinking by those involved in street scenes could be viewed, therefore, as a visible sign of social exclusion, whether chosen or not by the young people themselves. This scene's participants drank cheap beverage alcohol obtained from convenience stores and shops at petrol stations, the first group of adult stakeholders in the drinking scene. The second stakeholder group was the police. Young people felt threatened by the stigmatizing and excluding consequences associated with the intervention of this adult stakeholder group, although, in reality, the police often adopted the role of social workers by driving drunk youths home or calling rescue services.

The Disco Scene

The second typical type of youth alcohol scene was the disco scene, again named after the common meeting place. Young adults drinking in pubs or nightclubs were subsumed into this group. Participants of disco scenes were from varied social backgrounds but mostly belonged to the middle class and had enough money to frequent the fashionable youthful drinking places (with a predominantly young-adult clientele under 30 years old) from Thursdays to Sundays. The other days of the week were normally devoted to studying or work. The drinking places, especially the nightclubs, offered a multitude of bargains designed to attract young customers and satisfy their needs. Although the visitors of disco scenes reported less frequent alcohol consumption than members of street scenes, they drank to intoxication and engaged in fighting and nuisance-related misconduct at least as often. Drinking in disco scenes was a visible sign of social inclusion, and, if the young people became too drunk or disruptive, it was mostly private security employees who intervened. Troublemakers were thrown out of the venues, some being eventually picked up by the police.

The Private Scene

The third typical alcohol scene emerged in the course of the study: the private scene. It did not take place in a public drinking arena and so could not be directly observed. Key informants repeatedly mentioned heavy-drinking groups of young people from privileged social backgrounds who meet in private premises and are supplied with drinks by their parents. The private alcohol scene was largely out of the reach of police and private control agencies, even if its participants engaged in underage or harmful drinking. Participants of this scene became visible and attracted public attention only in extreme cases; but, contrary to the reaction to other alcohol scenes, that visibility did not arouse disapproval and even invoked a positive response. The most prominent example of a well-received conspicuous display of youthful drunkenness was the "party weeks" of Austrian high school students after graduation. (This fits with the transition festivities described earlier.) Annually, thousands of school graduates meet for 1 or more weeks in hotels at seaside resorts reserved for them (e.g., in Turkey). They celebrate by attending 24-hour parties, associated with heavy drinking but also fighting and some serious public nuisance; these youths are guarded by security and medical emergency personnel. Many such graduation journeys are sponsored by businesses (e.g., the media, sports, and banking industries) and are marketed through a daily newspaper. Media reports and images normally present a beautiful, successful, and promising young generation having fun. In a group discussion, however, this scene's participants drew a different picture. They talked about excessive drinking, risky sexual behavior, and assaults as much as about fun: "In the wider sense, the basic focus is on bottling each other, and on having sex. …"

Comparing the interactions between young people and stakeholders in the three alcohol scenes, Eisenbach-Stangl et al. (2008) found a number of ways in which the boundaries of drunkenness were shaped and, in particular, how public responses and sanctions were colored by sociodemographic factors that typified different youth groups. The research findings indicated the following:

- Accounts given by young people (interviewed individually and in groups) confirmed the authors' view that teachers did not play a role in shaping alcohol consumption and drunkenness, and that parents were "often fighting a losing battle."
- Parental efforts to shape the limits of drinking behavior were met with resistance and the firm conviction held by their children that, in Austria today, it is impossible to prevent anyone's choices about alcohol, regardless of the drinking age limits and other official regulations.

Adult stakeholder interventions varied widely depending on the type of the alcohol scene. This intensified the differences between the scenes and had implications for the social inclusion and exclusion of different segments of young people. For one youth subgroup, heavy drinking and drunkenness were publicly viewed as a deserved reward and associated with glamour and inclusion; for other subgroups, heavy drinking was branded as a nuisance and met with threats of further social exclusion and possible stigmatization through visible control measures. Furthermore, the authors suggested that, based on adult intervention approaches, the drinking context surrounding many young people may encourage drunkenness and exclude only those who transgress the generously drawn limits.

A similar picture of differential responses to drunken behavior among groups of young people comes from research carried out in Scotland.

Young People and Street Drinking in Scotland

In a study of 16- to 25-year-old Scottish street drinkers, Galloway et al. (2007) distinguished four subcultures and demonstrated how their drinking reflected not only their chosen group "image," but also the interaction between the groups and between the police and group members.

Neds was the term adopted by one group of young people to describe their distinctive culture, which conformed to the stereotypical image of neds as middle-class young people wearing casual sports clothes and gold jewelry. *Alternatives* were the young people who wore dark clothing and heavy makeup, had piercings and silver jewelry in "gothic" style, and conformed to a "punk" or "grunge" image. *Mainstream* youths did not have an identifiable subculture image; their dress style reflected "high street" fashion. The fourth category, *mixed* youths, mainly consisted of a combination of young people who were mainstream and alternative. Another factor distinguishing the groups from each other was the preferred alcohol beverage. In particular, the chosen drink of neds was Buckfast, associated with street drinkers and a macho image and disliked by the alternative and mainstream groups.

Both ned clothing and Buckfast symbolized a youth drinking culture seen as socially unacceptable and, therefore, attracting differential, sometimes unfair, treatment from the police. As one ned commented:

> Aye, that's what the police are looking for (indicates Buckfast). See when they start walking aboot this hill, they'll pick us out of the bunch coz we don't look like students. They don't like us being up here coz we're not students. (Galloway et al., 2007, p. 18)

Members of other groups agreed that similar behaviors elicited different public responses depending on the youth group and where the drinking was taking place rather than on how drunk they were or how they were behaving: (The police) " … targeted all the boys with, all the football boys in shorts and no tops, with the bottles of Buckfast, you know what I mean really, kind of classical drunk Glaswegian boy" (Galloway et al., 2007, p. 19).

In the course of the study, researchers themselves witnessed the differences in police procedures but concluded from their observations and interviews that police intervention roused defiance and that drinking habits remained the same, although neds in particular were likely to seek out more secluded locations for their activities.

As in other studies, outdoor drinking was seen by young people to have some advantages in that the drinkers were less physically and socially restricted. On the other hand, as Coleman and Cater (2005) found in their study of 14- to 17-year-olds in the United Kingdom, outdoor consumption in unsupervised locations was linked to a greater likelihood of drunkenness than drinking in more controlled settings. For many in the Scottish study (Galloway et al., 2007), outdoor drinking was a forced choice due to a number of factors—being underage or having underage friends, behaving in a way that had resulted in expulsion from indoor settings, and being "costed out" because drinking in pubs and nightclubs was too expensive. Police strategies, which included group dispersal, and neds' attempts to avoid police intervention by moving from one location to another meant that "[t]he high mobility of these groups increased the risk of violent territorial clashes with other youths in their local areas" (Galloway et al., 2007, p. 2). Again, the study illustrated how, in modern societies, the boundaries of drunkenness are differentially constructed depending on a multitude of factors.

Youthful Drunkenness: Elastic Boundaries

In the preceding accounts from Austria and Scotland, it is not argued that differential treatment is necessarily unwarranted on every occasion, only that similar types of drunken behaviors are more or less tolerated depending on a range of factors that serve to expand or contract the boundaries placed on drunkenness. Studies of young people's drinking illustrate the complexity of factors that shape modern drunkenness and the ways in which social and cultural differences interact with regulatory practices and public perceptions to set differential boundaries for different population groups. This is further explored in the U.K. context by Case Study 5.1 at the end of this chapter.

CONCLUSION

In this chapter, as in much of the available literature, there is a focus on research carried out in Europe and other Western countries where there are, perhaps, considerable commonalities in lifestyles, social structures, and belief systems. However, in considering the influences that shape modern youth drunkenness, we need to remind ourselves that, despite many commonalities, there are still enormous differences among regions, countries, and areas within countries. Factors such as gender, social status, ethnic group, and religion operate everywhere to determine whether and how people drink and what is seen as acceptable or a transgression of the formal and informal rules governing public behavior; all modern societies have ground rules regarding appropriate drinking, drunkenness occasions, and contexts when the boundaries are relaxed. But, as examples given earlier in the chapter illustrate, how behavior and its boundaries are defined is the outcome of a dynamic process that is subject to multiple variations, including social and cultural change beyond the individual, social, and economic drivers of alcohol consumption.

We have explored the extent to which traditional approaches to youth drunkenness survive and transcend generational change. There may be, as some have suggested, a real change in generational attitudes toward drunkenness, with young people adopting drinking patterns that go beyond the boundaries of traditional transition rituals and experimentation and herald a "new culture of intoxication." However, as Järvinen and Room (2007) pointed out in their review of youth drinking cultures, there continue to be social structures and norms protecting younger generations from a culture that accepts drinking to drunkenness. The question of whether there has been a real generational shift or mainly a shift in adult perceptions is still open to debate (Järvinen & Room, 2007, pp. 4–6).

CASE STUDY 5.1: How and Why Intoxication Features So Highly on the U.K. Political Agenda

Jean Coussins

The trouble with intoxication is that one person's pleasure is another person's pain. Furthermore, pleasure can turn into pain, although never the other way round. This book has taken a look at what people seek through intoxication, what they get, what they impose on others, and what society is prepared to do about it.

As discussed in Chapter 4, the United Kingdom has a long history of public and political debate about the degree to which alcohol consumption should be regulated. The consequences of drinking to excess lie at the heart of the dilemma about whether state intervention should attempt to punish or protect, or whether people should be free to damage themselves if they so choose. When it comes to damaging other people, however, for example, as a result of a drunken attack or alcohol-impaired driving, public consent to intervene is not at all equivocal—on the contrary. Thus, despite the United Kingdom having some of the most severe penalties for drinking and driving in Europe, a public opinion survey showed almost unanimous support for even heavier penalties for persistent offenders (MORI, 2001).

In the last 10 to 15 years, the issue of drunkenness, or "binge" drinking, has gathered social, political, and media momentum as never before. In many ways, it is a case of *plus ça change:* People will get drunk, especially young adults, and people will suffer and complain, but then people move on. In other ways, however, there have been some distinct (and sometimes contradictory) shifts. For many years, the government's nervousness at being branded the "nanny state" was one of the reasons it resisted demands to introduce restrictions on alcohol marketing and availability and even only half-heartedly promoted its own sensible drinking message. The persistence of the problem of binge drinking, however—both actual and perceived—has led to a markedly different attitude emerging, where concerns about public health, national reputation, the cost of alcohol misuse, and not a little moral panic have combined to strengthen the government's resolve that certain interventions are justified and, indeed, required from a responsible government, even one that espouses "light touch" regulation in other areas as a matter of principle. What are the shifts that have led to this change?

First, there has been a shift in the contexts and motivation for drunkenness, where young people with resources are captured by a new, commercially driven hedonistic culture of excess, in which alcohol plays a central part. By contrast, young people without resources or prospects use alcohol in much the same way as any other drug—to hide, escape, and forget. There is a world of difference between the group of 13- to 16-year-old "street drinkers," described in this chapter (see also Brain & Parker, 1997), and the young employed adults with significant disposable income who regard a drunken Friday night out as a normal social entitlement and at whom various industry and government campaigns have been targeted. Yet, both groups are motivated by drinking as a social event, and for both groups there is an explicit and deliberate objective of "getting off their heads," "buzzing," or drinking to feel disinhibited and more socially confident. It would be a mistake, however, to respond to these two groups in the same way. The underage youths are, by definition, doing something illicit and covert. They may well have broken the law by obtaining their alcohol in the first place, and although they might "have a laugh," their drinking episodes are "fuelled by a sense of despair or nihilism. In short, they had few other options for purchasing pleasure other than alcohol (or, for some, drugs) because of their own poverty and that of their immediate surroundings" (Brain & Parker, 1997, p. 64). Some researchers, like Brain and Parker (1997), conclude that heavy-handed policing of these young people would be counterproductive, and that the most helpful form of intervention would be to concentrate on inclusion and to apply moderate rather than zero tolerance.

The young adults aged between 18 and 24 years who display their intoxication through boisterous drunkenness, on the other hand, have a completely different mind-set. They are celebratory, overt, aggressive, and reckless as to the offense their behavior may cause to others. This group is responsible for a disproportionate amount of crime and disorder and, despite being in a minority among their peers, its members are so visible that their behavior appears to be "typical" to the public. Their visibility has also increased because of the physical changes in the landscape of licensed premises over the past decade, with local government authorities allowing greater concentrations of bars and nightclubs in town centers than ever before. Abundant and regular coverage in the tabloid media of the *Booze Britain** variety has encouraged this impression. The culture of excess has also been exported abroad, causing national shame, as these young adults have headed for resorts like Ibiza for their holidays, intent on indulging themselves in whatever excesses they like in public, including drink, drugs, and sex. At home, reality television shows like *Big Brother* have reinforced and promoted an attitude among this age group of regarding drunkenness as entertainment.

The result has been a public and political response calling for vigorous law enforcement, additional laws, and inclusion of new offenses into ordinances, such as the prohibition of alcohol consumption in certain public places, backed up by long-term public educational efforts by an alliance of government and nongovernmental stakeholders to change the drinking culture in which such behavior appears to be accepted, or at least expected. The entrenched culture around drunkenness in the United Kingdom was acknowledged in 1995 when the government amended its sensible-drinking guidelines from a weekly limit (21 8 g units for men, 14 for women) to daily benchmarks (3–4 units for men, 2–3 for women). This was because it was thought that too many people were misinterpreting the weekly limits as permitting the consumption of the whole week's units in one event on a Friday or Saturday night. The government realized it needed to be clearer and, in particular, express the guidelines in a way that explicitly discouraged drunkenness. More than a decade later, the government's latest alcohol harm reduction strategy identified 18- to 24-year-old "binge drinkers" as one of the top priorities for the effort now required "to challenge the belief that drunkenness and antisocial behaviour are an accepted part of an English 'drinking culture'" (Department of Health, Home Office, Department for Education and Skills, & Department for Culture, Media and Sport, 2007, p. 47). In canvasing public opinion, the government found that views are changing: "Most of us now think that the social attitude to 'crossing the line' between having a good time to putting ourselves and others at risk needs to change" (p. 57).

* *Booze Britain* is a "fly-on-the-wall" British television show; each episode follows groups of friends on their heavy-drinking outings in various U.K. cities and towns and teams of paramedics called in to respond to problems.

There is a fresh commitment to sustained national campaigning that will target not only the excessive drinkers themselves, but also public tolerance of drunks and drunkenness. Significantly, the strategy aims not only to discourage excessive drinking, but at the same time positively reinforce and promote sensible drinking, which, it is acknowledged, is what most people actually do.

The second clear shift concerns the culprit held accountable, with the finger of blame being directed unswervingly at the industry. Producers and brands are accused of encouraging and glamorizing excessive drinking through their advertising and promotions. Pubs and nightclubs stand accused of ignoring the law prohibiting the sale of alcohol to intoxicated customers. Supermarkets are currently under serious scrutiny for the way in which their pricing policies, in particular deep discounting, could lead to increased binge drinking. Of course, there may well be room for improvement in industry behavior, although compliance with the strict—and recently further strengthened—advertising code rules is high (Sinclair, 2009).

A corollary of the focus on industry behavior, however, seems to have been a downgrading of the notion of personal responsibility. Indeed, a report from the Nuffield Council on Bioethics (2007), which examined ethics across a range of public health issues including alcohol, concluded that reliance on personal behavior to influence public health outcomes is "too simplistic." Instead, a new stewardship model was proposed, based on a sliding scale of intervention depending on the level of threat to population health and a carefully argued analysis of the balance between individual liberty and the public good. In relation to alcohol consumption, the authors concluded that the government strategy falls short, and that more coercive measures are warranted to restrict and control price, marketing, and availability.

Underlying both these shifts is the war of statistics. Never has there been an issue better able to demonstrate the refrain that you can prove anything with statistics than the issue of alcohol consumption! Their selective use is employed by the promoters of intervention and of self-regulation. It is true that the United Kingdom has one of the highest incidences of youth drunkenness in Europe. It is also true that the number of 11- to 15-year-olds who drink has declined, and that the number of teenage abstainers is higher than ever before. It is true that among 16- to 24-year-olds, nearly a third of men and over a fifth of women are drinking at harmful levels. It is also true that harmful drinking in this and all other age groups has decreased significantly since 2003. It is true that 18- to 24-year-olds who binge drink are far more likely to admit to criminal or disorderly conduct than regular drinkers in the same age group. It is also true that offenses committed by those under the influence of alcohol have dropped by about a third since 1995.

The juxtaposition of alarmist and encouraging figures could go on and on. The question is whether the government, the industry, and everyone else adversely affected by the harmful social consequences of drunkenness have the nerve, the commitment, and the resources to pursue and sustain the effort to achieve long-term, lasting culture change, as well as supporting strong law enforcement in the immediate term. If not, the danger is that quick-fix measures such as advertising restrictions will in practice contribute to that most undesirable of social outcomes for intoxication—drive it underground, all the more glamorous and attractive for being illicit, and well beyond the influence of a balanced regime of legitimate social and legal controls.

REFERENCES

Beccaria, F., & Sande, A. (2003). Drinking games and rite of life projects: A social comparison of the meaning and functions of young people's use of alcohol during the rite of passage to adulthood in Italy and Norway. *Young, 11*, 99–119.

Brain, K., & Parker, H. (1997). *Drinking with design: Alcopops, designer drinks and youth culture.* London: Portman Group.

Chatterton, P., & Hollands, R. (2001). *Changing our "toon": Youth, nightlife and urban change in Newcastle.* Newcastle upon Tyne, UK: Newcastle University Press.

Coleman, L., & Cater, S. (2005). *Underage "risky" drinking: Motivations and outcomes.* York, UK: Joseph Rowntree Foundation.

Department of Health, Home Office, Department for Education and Skills, & Department for Culture, Media and Sport. (2007). *Safe. Sensible. Social: The next steps in the National Alcohol Strategy.* London: Home Office.

Eisenbach-Stangl, I., Bernardis, A., Fellöcker, K., Haberhauer-Stidl, J., & Schmied, G. (2008). *Jugendliche Alkoholszenen. Konsumkontexte, Trinkmotive, Prävention.* [Youth alcohol scenes: Consumption contexts, drinking motives, prevention] Vienna, Austria: European Centre for Social Welfare Policy and Research.

Galloway, J., Forsyth, A., & Shewan, D. (2007, February). *Young people's street drinking behaviour: Investigating the influence of marketing and subculture.* London: Glasgow Centre for the Study of Violence.

Gómez Fraguela, J. A., Fernández Pérez, N., Romero Triñanes, E., & Luengo Martín, A. (2008). El botellón y el consumo de alcohol y otras drogas en la juventud [*Botellón* and consumption of alcohol and other drugs in youth]. *Psicothema, 20,* 211–217.

Graham, K., & Homel, R. (1997). Creating safer bars. In M. Plant, E. Single, & T. Stockwell (Eds.), *Alcohol: Minimising the harm. What works?* (pp. 171–192). London: Free Association Books.

Graham, K., & Homel, R. (2008). *Raising the bar: Preventing aggression in and around bars, pubs and clubs.* Devon, UK: Willan.

Hadfield, P. (2006). *Bar wars: Contesting the night in contemporary British cities.* Oxford, UK: Oxford University Press.

Harnett, R., Thom, B., Herring, R., & Kelly, M. (2000). Alcohol in transition: Towards a model of young men's drinking styles. *Journal of Youth Studies, 3,* 61–77.

Heath, D. B. (2000). *Drinking occasions: Comparative perspectives on alcohol and culture.* Philadelphia: Brunner Mazel.

Heley, J. (2008). Rounds, Range Rovers and rurality: The drinking geographies of a New Squirearchy. *Drugs: Education, Prevention and Policy, 15,* 315–321.

Järvinen, M., & Room, R. (Eds.). (2007). *Youth drinking cultures: European experiences.* Aldershot, UK: Ashgate.

Jayne, M., Valentine, G., & Holloway, S. L. (2008a) Fluid boundaries—British binge drinking and European civility: Alcohol and the production and consumption of public space. *Space & Polity, 12,* 81–100.

Jayne, M., Valentine, G., & Holloway, S. L. (2008b). Geographies of alcohol, drinking and drunkenness: A review of progress. *Progress in Human Geography, 32,* 247–263.

Jayne, M., Valentine, G., & Holloway, S. L. (2008c). The place of drink: Geographical contributions to alcohol studies. *Drugs: Education, Prevention and Policy, 15,* 219–232.

Martinic, M., & Measham, F. (Eds.). (2008). *Swimming with crocodiles: The culture of extreme drinking.* New York: Routledge.

Mastache, C., Mistral, W., Velleman, R., & Templeton, L. (2008). Partnership working in community alcohol prevention programs. *Drugs: Education, Prevention and Policy, 15*(Suppl. 1), 4–14.

Midford, R., Wayte, K., Catalano, P., Gupta, R., & Chikritzhs, T. (2005). The legacy of a community mobilisation project to reduce alcohol related harm. *Drug and Alcohol Review, 24,* 3–11.

Mistral, W., Velleman, R., Mastache, C., & Templeton, L. (2007, October). *UKCAPP: An evaluation of 3 U.K. community alcohol prevention programmes.* London: Alcohol Education and Research Council.

MORI. (2001). *Alcohol and society.* London: Portman Group.

Nuffield Council on Bioethics. (2007). *Public health: Ethical issues.* Cambridge, UK: Author.

Parker, H., Aldridge, J., & Measham, F. (1998). *Illegal leisure: The normalization of adolescent recreational drug use.* London: Routledge.

Parliamentary Office of Science and Technology. (2005, July). Binge drinking and public health. *Postnote, 244,* 1–4. Retrieved November 30, 2009, from http://www.parliament.uk/documents/upload/postpn244.pdf

Rodrigues-Martos, A. (2006). The Spanish *botellón,* a particular way of bingeing. *Nordic Studies on Alcohol and Drugs, 23,* 137–142.

Sadounig, D. (2008). *Komatrinken in den Medien: Ein Zerrbild* [Coma drinking in the media: A distorted image]. Unpublished manuscript, Vienna, Austria.

Sinclair, R. (2009). Marketing beverage alcohol. In M. Grant & M. Leverton (Eds.), *Working together to reduce harmful drinking* (pp. 63–90). New York: Routledge.

The Stationery Office. (2003). *Licensing Act 2003.* Retrieved September 30, 2009, from http://www.opsi.gov.uk/acts/acts2003/pdf/ukpga_20030017_en.pdf

The Stationery Office. (2005). *Licences and licensing: The Licensing Act 2003 (transitional provisions)* (Order 2005 No. 40). Retrieved September 30, 2009, from http://www.opsi.gov.uk/SI/si2005/20050040.htm#n1

Thom, B. (2007). Alcohol: Protecting the young, protecting society. In B. Thom, R. Sales, & J. J. Pearce (Eds.), *Growing up with risk* (pp. 241–258). Bristol, UK: Policy Press.

Uhl, A., & Kobrna, U. (2008). *Kurzexpertise zu: Jugendschutz in Österreich—alkoholspezifische Bestimmungen* [A short review of: Protection of children and young people in Austria—Alcohol-specific regulations]. Unpublished manuscript, Vienna, Austria.

van Gennep, A. (2004). *The rites of passage.* London: Routledge. (Original work published 1909)

World Health Organization Regional Office for Europe. (2001). *Declaration on young people and alcohol.* Retrieved September 30, 2009, from http://www.euro.who.int/AboutWHO/Policy/20030204_1

6

Concluding Remarks

Trish Worth

This book approaches an age-old phenomenon—drunkenness—from a fresh and interdisciplinary perspective. "Expressions of drunkenness" have, indeed, been embedded in societies and cultures around the world for centuries. Such expressions also support the assertion that there is a distinction between *intoxication* and *drunkenness*. For example, someone who is drinking might be described as "blotto" or "plastered" because of his or her drunken behavior (versus biological intoxication), and people who are intoxicated yet do not exhibit overtly drunken behavior might be described as having "a hollow leg" or being able to "hold their liquor." Moreover, when examined comprehensively from biological, cultural, and social perspectives, it becomes clear that intoxication typically refers to a physiological state, whereas drunkenness points to actions and social effects often associated with intoxication.

Why the focus on such a distinction? For those who participated in the 2007 workshop and later served as authors of this book (see Chapter 1), this point emerged as a helpful first step in determining practical solutions to reduce problems from intoxicated and drunken behavior. If we are to achieve long-term, self-sustaining cultural change, we must first have sufficient understanding of the individual and collective meanings, aims, and functions of drunkenness. In particular, it is important to understand the factors that underpin patterns of drinking and shape potential outcomes. For example, although some drinking patterns will contribute to increased risk for negative health and social outcomes, there is also considerable research evidence that moderate drinking can reduce the risk of heart disease and, although not risk-free, is associated with lower overall mortality than abstinence or heavy drinking.

As we established in the preceding chapters, a multitude of factors have been shown to influence drinking patterns—from population-specific characteristics (e.g., gender, age, socioeconomics, and genetics) to the drinking context (e.g., culture and drinking settings), to beliefs about alcohol and leisure and the extent to which drunkenness is tolerated within a community. Generally speaking, in many societies, there is now heightened awareness of the social and health issues associated with intoxication. Numerous efforts have been launched in support of a shift in drinking cultures that would discourage excess and encourage responsibility. We hope to have helped lend insight to such efforts by communicating about cultural nuances and societal norms and the realities of issues we face in efforts to reduce alcohol-related harm, as well as encourage the responsible enjoyment of beverage alcohol.

If, as our authors assert, the terms *intoxication* and *drunkenness* are separate yet interrelated, we can gain actionable insight into these phenomena. For instance, if intoxication is more of a physiological state compared to drunkenness, which speaks more to behavior and cultural norms, we can then approach issues and consequences related to both phenomena in the appropriate context, understanding that they exist on continuums. However a culture interprets drunkenness—whether it is attached to an age-old concept such as "400 rabbits" or another aspect of cultural context—a society's commonly held perceptions of alcohol and drunken behavior are critical aspects of this analysis. Although we do not arrive at a neat and tidy universal definition of drunkenness, by bringing existing definitions together and exploring their meanings and commonalities, we are able to offer language and conceptual tools to help advance the ongoing discussion and inform the debate.

Index

F

G

H

I

J

K

L

M

N

O

P

Y